THIS BOOK IS DEDICATED AS A LABOUR OF LOVE TO MY BEAUTIFUL FRIENDS WHO HAVE SHOWN ME JOY AND ACCEPTANCE AND HAVE PUT ME BACK TOGETHER WHEN I NEEDED IT. TO FI WHO WAS BRAVE, WOOLIE WHO SHOWED ME THE POWER OF CRYSTALS, AND SUKEY (MY CONFIDANT, CONSPIRATOR, CONSILERI AND SISTER) THERE ARE NO WORDS TO WHAT YOU HAVE BROUGHT TO MY LIFE. TO ALL THOSE WHO INSPIRE ME TO FIND THE LAUGHTER IN SMALL MOMENTS AND THAT TIME WITH PEOPLE WE LOVE IS INDEED THE MOST PRECIOUS THING WE HAVE.............

AND LASTLY...FOR MEGAN C AND ALL THE OTHERS OUT THERE FOR WHOM THIS BOOK IS INTENDED.

# HELLO THERE,

My name is Lucy Wise and I am a Clinical Psychologist who has worked for over 20 years in the field of trauma and mental health but I have also worked with those going through cancer treatment. I have also had the experience of friends who have battled the big C (some who lost the fight and some who won) and as a support person I have seen the good, bad and ugly and the impact on families and those who love the person suffering through treatment. A cancer diagnosis is traumatic for you and also those around you. A good mental headspace can help with what you are going to have to go through as part of your treatment. I am sorry that you are going to have to face this difficult battle and I wish from the bottom of my heart you didn't have to. Yes the word "cancer" it is terrible and awful and terrifying but now that you are facing it, this book is here to help you find some ways to cope. Working your way through the book won't make it less awful but it can help you have a pathway and road map to get through it and get out the other side. While this book encourages you to follow medical advice it also gives you an outlet for the trauma and distress associated with your diagnosis. I wrote this book because I was frustrated that I could not find something for my patients and friends who needed help at the point of diagnosis before they were able see a therapist to process all of the chaos of a diagnosis. I had written a book prior to this one about trauma but my friend was diagnosed with cancer and it made me realise the huge gap between the diagnosis of cancer and being able to get help. What someone really needs is help and strategies "right now". My friend insisted that I write this book for her and others.....so I did!

Please take advantage of this workbook. This book is designed to assist you to develop skills to manage your symptoms, provide you with information and help you construct strategies for when you need them. These skills are resources that you may need in the future and it is designed to compliment your individual therapy. This book is designed to help you as part of your journey with lots of ideas and strategies for you to consider. This book is however not a replacement for a good therapist who can help guide you and provide professional help while you are undergoing treatment.

Work through the book over the next couple of weeks and add to it as you feel necessary. Whenever you need these resources in the future they will be available to you here in this workbook safely stored in one place. You will notice there are normal looking pages and some pages have coloured sections on them for you to write in.

The most important part of this book is the cover. I didn't know before I started this book why Daffodils were associated with Cancer. I now know that it is because they bloom after winter.

# TABLE OF CONTENTS

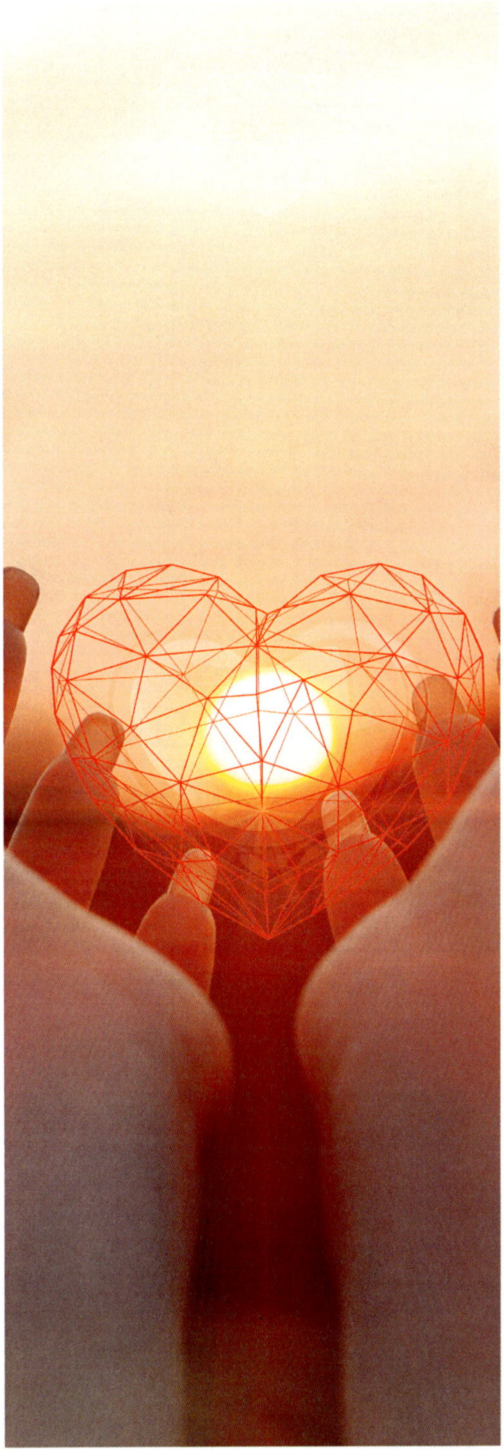

# MY ROAD MAP

1. **UNDERSTNADING MY DIAGNOSIS**

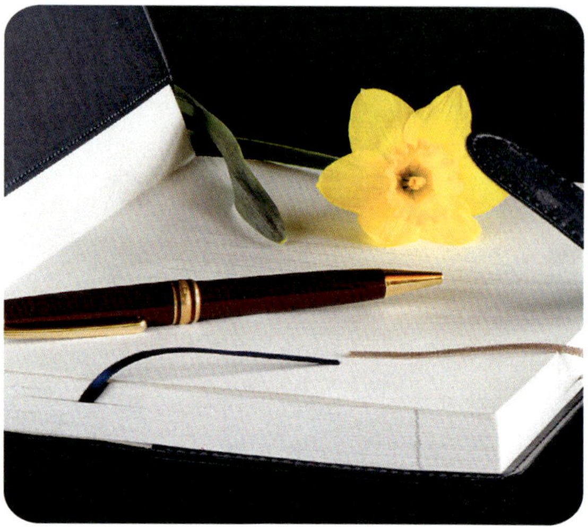

2. Education about PTSD and trauma associated with your diagnosis and related conditions.

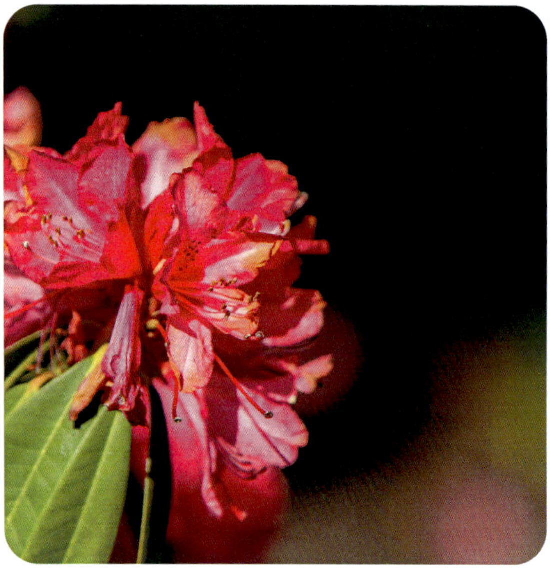

3. STRATEGIES TO MANAGE YOUR SYMPTOMS INCLUDING SUPPORTS

4. Trauma focussed therapy (confronting the painful memories, associations and feared situations including medical treatments)

5. COGNITIVE RESTRUCTURING

6. **Relapse prevention and ongoing support,**

7. **Sealed Section (only open this when you are ready or if you have too)**

# DIAGNOSIS

A diagnosis is isolating and can make us feel like we are the only people in the world. Traumatic events such as a cancer diagnosis are extremely threatening and can be totally overwhelming. A diagnosis can make us feel disconnected from those around us and very frightened. While it may feel at times hopeless..........you are hopefully seeking treatment and listening to the advice and recommendations from your doctors. However, you need to also think about your psychological health and how you are going to "get into the right headspace". With the right treatment there is hope and those who have a good outlook have a much better outcome and response to treatment. It is ok to recognise that your emotions are spiralling right now but with the right game plan you can lead the kind of life you want to lead while going through treatment and have the relationships you want to have.....even when walking the path you are on right now.

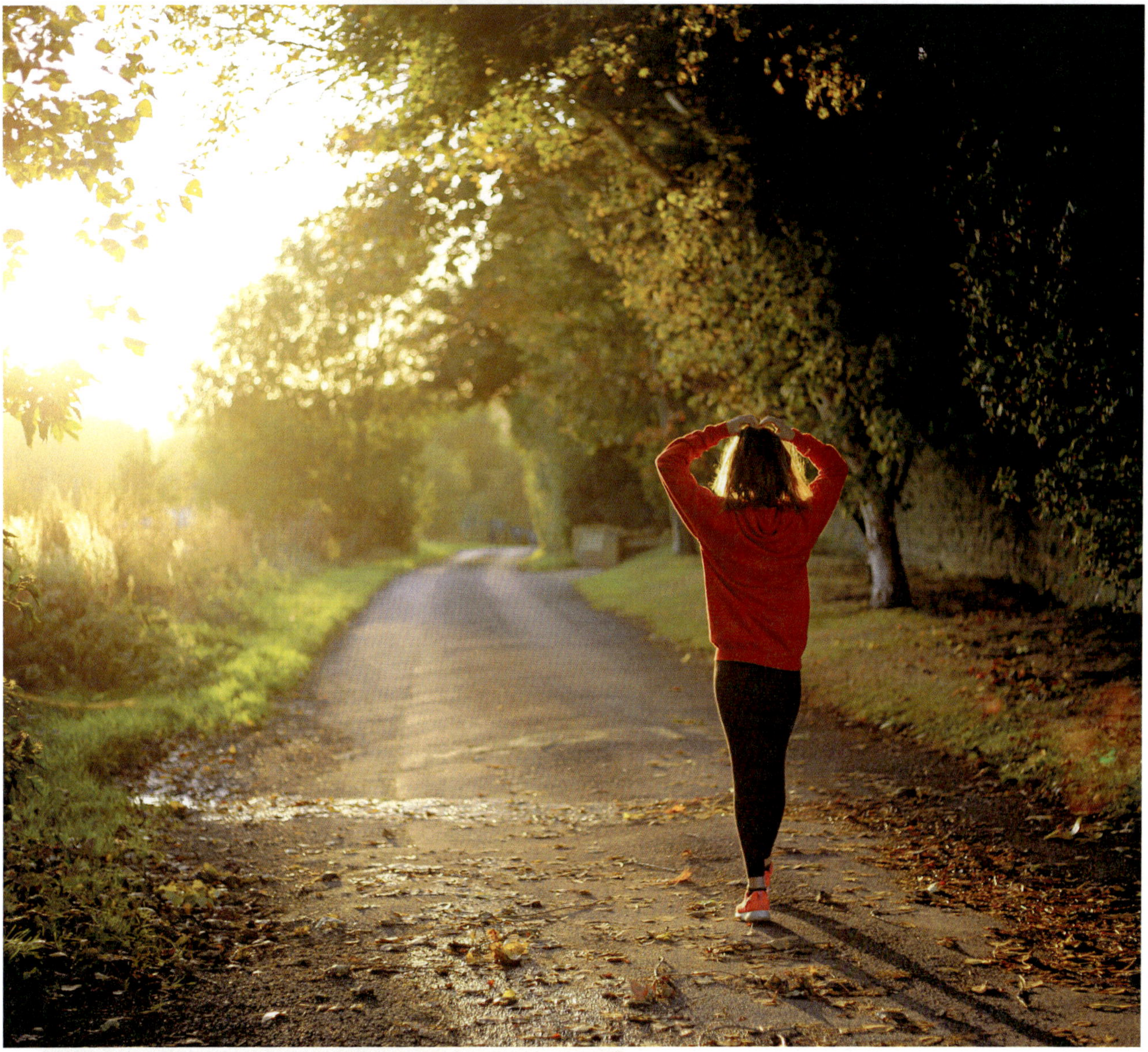

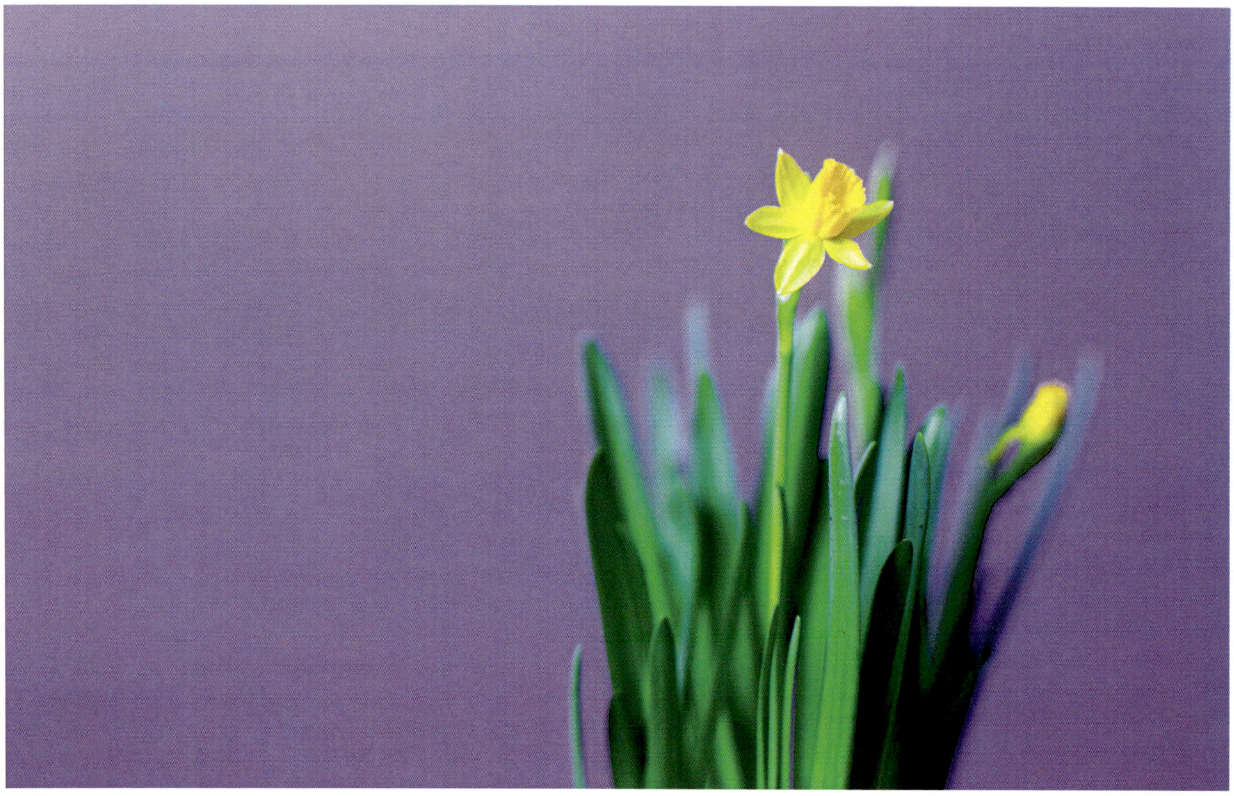

# TREATMENT AND RECOVERY

You have already started the first stage of managing in your emotions by acknowledging that your reactions to the traumatic event may not be healthy. You have also hopefully taken the step of seeking appropriate treatment from a mental health professional not to mention your medical team. Getting help is often frightening - for many, it is a leap into the unknown - but trying to recover from the trauma of this on your own is extremely difficult. It is important to remember that treatment can be painful and at times very hard work. Unfortunately, there is no easy way to get rid of the associations, triggers and memories or make them less distressing. There is no magic wand that your therapist or doctor can wave or tablet that you can take to make it all go away.....I wish it was that simple! The long-term gains of therapy can be enormous, giving you the opportunity to live your best life......even with cancer.

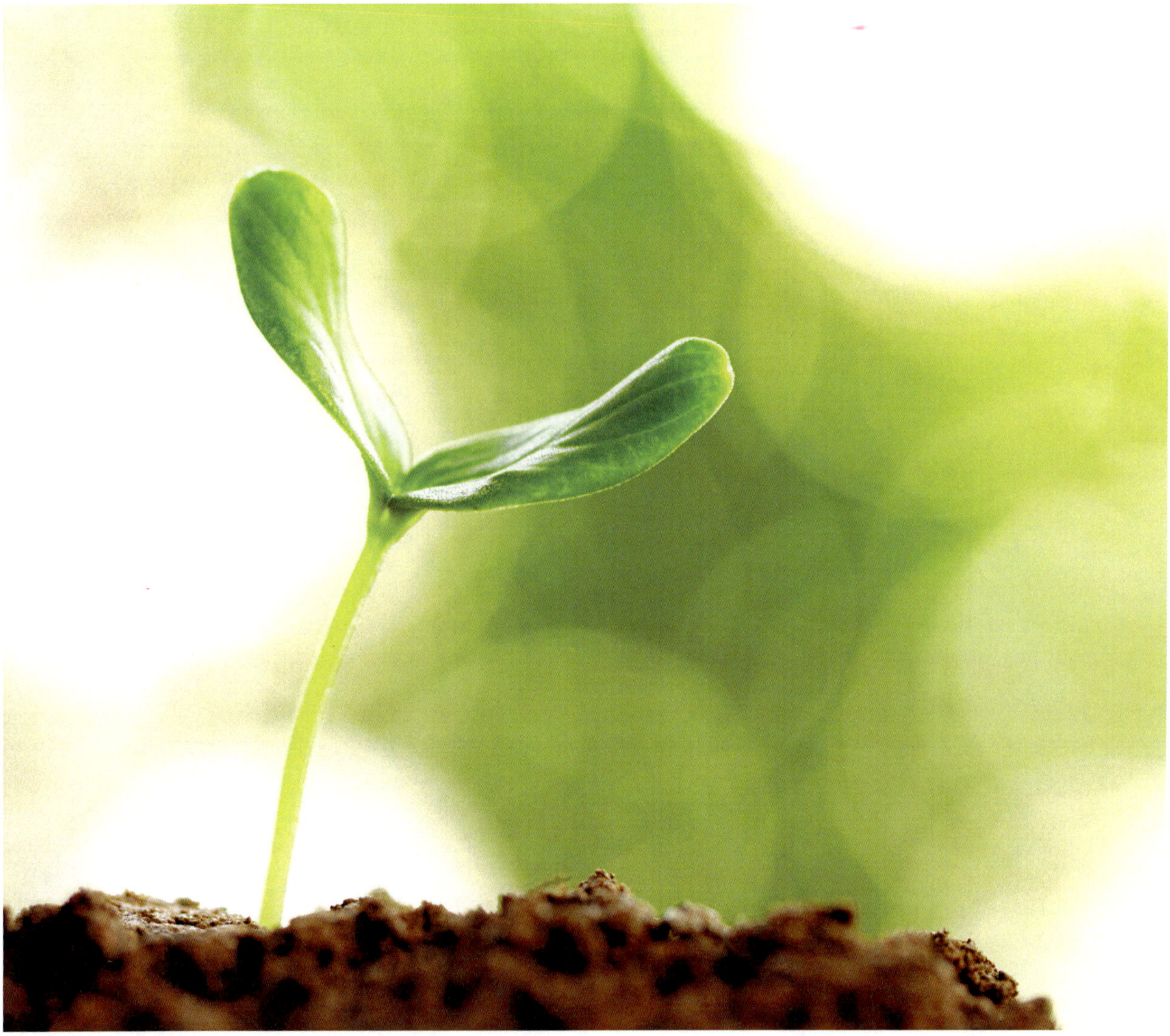

# WHERE DO I START?

Over the next few pages are a list of things for you to start to consider. There are a list of things for you to ask your doctors and things for you to be mindful of as part of your next steps. The list of questions provided are not there to help you challenge your specialists and recommended treatment, but rather they are a suggested starting point. They are some ideas of what you might need to ask your doctors (GP and Specialist) and hopefully help you feel a bit less out of control and are able to start to navigate some very foreign territory.

# WHAT DO I NEED TO KNOW?

Understanding cancer treatment can help you and your loved ones make informed decisions, manage expectations, and cope with the challenges of the treatment process. It is important to get good advice and if possible talk to others who have been through it. While the internet is a great source of information it is not necessarily the most accurate information. You want to try and be balanced in the information you get and certainly be careful and wary of weird websites promising a miracle cure or give you some dodgy advice that could cause pointless fear and anxiety! Here are some key points that you should consider and be prepared for about cancer treatment:

1. **Multidisciplinary Approach:** Cancer treatment often involves a multidisciplinary team of healthcare professionals, including oncologists, surgeons, radiation oncologists, nurses, and other specialists. This team collaborates to develop a comprehensive treatment plan tailored to the individual needs of each patient.
2. **Types of Treatment:** Cancer treatment may include various modalities, depending on the type, stage, and location of the cancer. Common treatment options include surgery, chemotherapy, radiation therapy, immunotherapy, targeted therapy, hormone therapy, stem cell transplant, and precision medicine approaches.
3. **Goals of Treatment:** The goals of cancer treatment vary depending on the specific circumstances of each patient. Treatment may be aimed at curing the cancer, controlling its growth and spread, relieving symptoms and improving quality of life (palliative care), or a combination of these goals.
4. **Treatment Planning:** Cancer treatment plans are personalized based on factors such as the type and stage of cancer, the patient's overall health and preferences, and the potential risks and benefits of treatment options. Patients should be actively involved in the decision-making process and have the opportunity to discuss treatment goals, options, and concerns with their healthcare team.
5. **Side Effects:** Cancer treatment can cause side effects that vary depending on the type of treatment and individual factors. Common side effects may include fatigue, nausea, vomiting, hair loss, changes in appetite, pain, neuropathy, and immune suppression. Not everyone experiences these side effects but it is important to be prepared for what you might expect from you treatment regime. Some side effects may be temporary and resolve after treatment, while others may persist or require supportive care.
6. **Supportive Care:** Supportive care plays a crucial role in cancer treatment by managing side effects, improving quality of life, and addressing the physical, emotional, and practical needs of patients and their families. Supportive care services may include pain management, nutrition counselling, psychosocial support, integrative therapies, rehabilitation, and palliative care.
7. **Follow-Up Care:** After completing active cancer treatment, patients typically require ongoing monitoring and follow-up care to monitor for recurrence, manage

late effects of treatment, and address survivorship issues. Follow-up care may include regular check-ups, imaging tests, blood tests, and screenings based on individual risk factors and guidelines.

8. **Clinical Trials:** Clinical trials are research studies that evaluate new cancer treatments, therapies, and interventions. Participating in a clinical trial may offer access to innovative treatments and contribute to the advancement of cancer care. Patients may discuss with their healthcare team whether participating in a clinical trial is a suitable option for them. There are pros and cons with clinical trials but it is worth asking your doctor what the options are and being informed.
9. **Coping Strategies:** Coping with cancer treatment involves developing strategies to manage physical symptoms, emotional distress, and practical challenges. Patients and their families may benefit from support groups, counselling, relaxation techniques, stress management, exercise, nutrition, and other self-care practices to promote overall well-being during treatment. Strategies will help both you and your support crew....this fight needs to be a "team effort".
10. **Communication:** Open and honest communication with healthcare providers, family members, and friends is essential throughout the cancer treatment process. Patients should feel able to ask questions, express concerns, and seek information and support from their healthcare team and support network.

This is time for you to start to educate yourself about the type of cancer, the treatment you are going to have and what to expect at each stage of your treatment program. For some of you there may only be a few side effects from treatment and for others the treatment regimes you need and the drugs used to "treat" your cancer can cause some pretty awful side effects. Regardless as you go through your treatment there will be days you will feel pretty tired and emotional and you will possibly have no energy or crave weird foods....anything can happen! However, it is important to know what to expect and so by educating yourself you will give yourself a better idea of what is coming in the next few months and also to be aware that you won't necessarily feel bad all the time but you are preparing for the days you might.

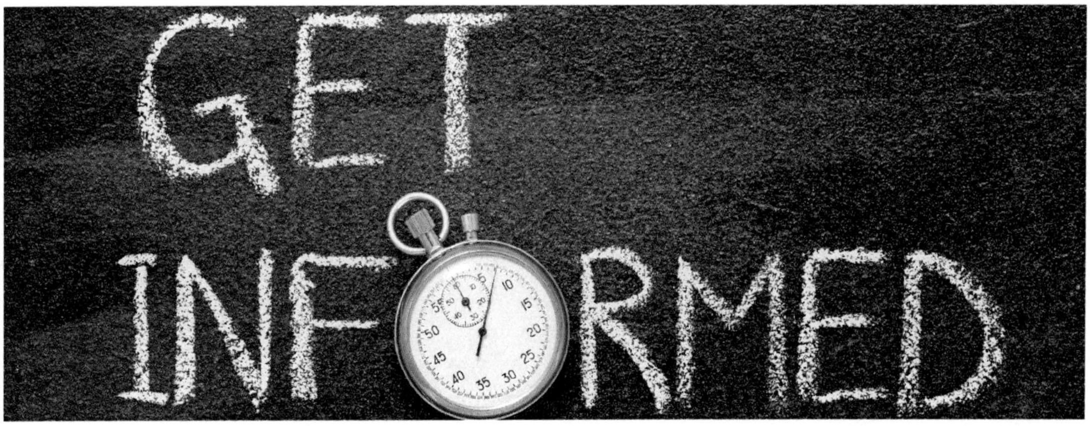

# QUESTION TIME!

When diagnosed with cancer, it's crucial to communicate effectively with your healthcare team to gather all necessary information, understand your treatment options, and make informed decisions. Before we go any further you can take a minute and try to get your head around all of the confusing things that are happening to you since you got the news that you have been diagnosed with cancer. You have now probably started a whirlwind of talking to people who are new to you and yet they have a lot of control over what happens to you, your body and what happens to you.  In the next few months you will be required to make lots of decisions and also choices that you never thought you would have to make. Take a minute and start to think about the sorts of questions you may need to ask. This is your body and you have a right to know what is going to happen next. Take the time to sit down and write some questions for your doctor in the space provided on the next page. Some key questions to ask your doctor or treating team that may help you understand what is going to happen next may include:

1. **What type and stage of cancer do I have?** Understanding the type and stage of cancer is fundamental to making informed decisions about treatment and prognosis.
2. **What are my treatment options?** Ask about the available treatment modalities, including surgery, chemotherapy, radiation therapy, immunotherapy, targeted therapy, or clinical trials. Also what are these treatments and what do they do?
3. **What are the goals of treatment?** Discuss whether the aim of treatment is curative versus remission, palliative, or aimed at symptom management.
4. **What are the potential side effects of treatment?** Understanding potential side effects can help you prepare for and manage treatment-related challenges.
5. **How will treatment affect my daily life?** Discuss the impact of treatment on daily activities, work, family, and other responsibilities.
6. **What supportive care services are available?** Ask about supportive care services such as nutrition counselling, pain management, psychological support, and integrative therapies. Ask if any of these people may be worth getting in contact with as key supports?
7. **Are there any complementary or alternative treatments I should consider?** Discuss whether complementary or alternative therapies may be appropriate to incorporate alongside conventional treatment. This might include diet and exercise. Exercise has been shown to have good health benefits even when people are undergoing chemotherapy.
8. **What is the prognosis?** While it can be challenging to predict outcomes, understanding the prognosis can help you plan for the future and make important decisions. This is a difficult question to ask as no one likes to think the worst.
9. **What clinical trials are available to me?** Ask about any ongoing clinical trials that may offer access to experimental treatments or new approaches to care. A clinical

trial is a research study that is conducted with patients to develop new treatments. There is an eligibility criteria and it is worth asking if you may be eligible and what are the conditions of being accepted into the trial. However, this also brings up new questions as you will need to think about where the study is based and will this delay your current treatment?

10. **What lifestyle changes can I make to support my treatment and recovery?**
    Discuss lifestyle modifications such as diet, exercise, smoking cessation, and stress management that may support your overall health and well-being. You need to be in the best place possible to give yourself the best chance of recovery.
11. **How frequently will I need follow-up appointments and monitoring?**
    Understand the schedule for follow-up appointments, tests, and surveillance to monitor for complications or treatment efficacy. There will be a lot of appointments and it is important that you have a clear understanding of what the schedule might be. Also ask how often you might see your specialist? How often are your appointments? Where are the appointments held? Is the doctor going away and if they do will someone else be involved in your care? Who are they? You may see an alternate doctor if your doctor is away and it is worth asking who this person might be so you are prepared and whether or not they may alter your current treatment protocol.
12. **How can I reach you (your doctor) if I have questions or concerns between appointments?**
    Ensure you have clear communication channels with your healthcare team and know who your contact people are if you are worried or if something is not right. What are the key phone numbers that you might need to call if you are worried?
13. **Initially you may (be in shock and) not want to know too much about your diagnosis.**
    Choosing to trust your doctor to make the best medical decisions for you is very confronting especially if you have only just met them this morning! While no one likes to be out of control and to be part of a system that "swings into action" around your treatment as you progress through your treatment the information you need to be aware of will naturally evolve. Be mindful that once the diagnosis is made then things start to happen very quickly.

Remember to take notes during your appointments with your medical team or bring a trusted friend or family member to help you remember the key information discussed in your appointments. I can't stress this enough, you may not remember key things as you could be in shock and only take in half of the information given to you. Don't hesitate to ask for clarification if you don't understand something or if the doctor uses words that sound bizarre. No, you are not stupid, these words are familiar to the doctor not you and you have probably never heard them before in your life. You are allowed to ask questions after all it is your body. Effective communication with your healthcare team is essential for navigating your cancer journey and make the most informed decisions about your care.

## NOTES AND QUESTIONS TO ASK THE DOCTOR OR SPECIALIST

# IT'S ABOUT ME!!!

Now is the time to consider some other things. These are practical things before we get into how to cope with emotions. As a clinician I have been used to talking to people about these next few issues when they are recently diagnosed and about to start cancer treatment. Often people don't know how or what they should be planning ahead for when they are undergoing treatment.

1. **Do you have income protection?:** Lets face it you may not be able to work as you undergo treatment, some people can but some can't, it will depend on your treatment regime. Income protection insurance can be particularly important for individuals diagnosed with cancer, as the illness may result in being unable to work for an extended period due to treatment, recovery, or ongoing health challenges. Income protection provides a source of income if you are unable to work and it can help cover essential expenses such as mortgage or rental payments, bills and medical costs. You may also need to check how long the waiting period is or what sorts of documentation you may need to provide to your insurance company. Double check as income protection may be part of your retirement benefits fund or you may have had a separate policy and sometimes it can be part of a life insurance policy called major illness and injury. Also check how much sick leave you have if you are employed as you may/will also need to use this while you are undergoing treatment as there are days you might be be able to work. Check how many hours of sick leave you have stored up. Now is the time to use them!
2. **I have a pet?:** Think about how you will look after your dog/cat/guinea pig or fish (or any other pet) when you may need to be in hospital. Can you put aside food for them or buy in bulk if people are willing to feed them while you are in hospital? Do you need to consider putting them in a kennel for a few days at a time when you are having treatment?
3. **Who do I need to tell about my diagnosis?:** This is different for friends and family which we will discuss soon. This is more practical and think about telling your children's teachers or school or how you would tell your employer? Some key people will need to know as you may need some extra help or some time off to have treatment and don't forget recovery time. Also consider how much you want them to know. In the case of the children's school for example it may impact on sporting activities and the school need to provide some extra support to the children.
4. **How much money do you have in the bank and what bills can be set up to be automatically paid?:** You are going to feel pretty awful for a while so think about all the ways you can reduce your stress and make sure life can continue without you having to experience additional unnecessary worry.
5. **What have you got booked in?:** Check what is booked and what can be moved. Right now you have a few things to worry about and that holiday to Fiji might need to be put off for a bit.
6. **Start putting food away in the freezer:** Yes people will want to help and you might need to buy a second freezer for all the casseroles! If you are alone or live by

yourself stockpiling food for days when you are struggling is a good idea. Do it now before things get really busy. Also consider what sort of food you might like and if people offer to help they mean well and in my experience they want to help to make life easier for you. If you feel like accepting help then perhaps give people some ideas of what you might like such as biscuits for the family or curry for a dinner (there is no point people giving you 200 lasagnes if you hate it).

7. **Photos:** Something a friend of mine said after her first round of treatment was she wished she had taken some lovely photos of herself before she got really ill. She said it wasn't because she was about the "doom" but more because she wanted photos of how she looked prior to having chemotherapy. This is something that really stuck with me as a therapist and friend. If you can, take some beautiful photos of you and your family or loved ones, even if your loved one is a pet (fur family). These photos will be there so that you have something to look at when you are having treatment as you may look different after treatment. This is something that isn't often openly discussed and it can be very confronting for those involved as it can have a very "dark overtone" but these photos of you will be very special to those who love you and also to you. How many times do we as parents or partners take a picture of others in the family but rarely are we all in the picture. If you can get a friend to take photos or get some professionally taken. Make it a fun day and celebrate you with your family and friends. These will be very special memories. We did this with a friend of mine who got her cancer diagnosis but just prior to treatment starting and then after we took the photos we all celebrated with a glass or two of Champagne! It's a day I will never forget.
8. **Journal:** This is something to consider. It is personal and some people want to do this and others do not. This is your call.....if you do want to journal consider the type of journal and what you want to put in it. It might be a bullet journal or you may want to put things down that you are worried about. It might also be a time to write down things for people who love you such as favourite recipes. You don't need to look at this as "doom" but these are ideas and thoughts that once treatment has finished you may be able to carry out that holiday to Iceland to walk on the black beaches, teach your granddaughter to line dance or cuddle a baby Orangutan or say the important messages to those people who are close to you.
9. **Do I need a house keeper?:** This will depend on your circumstances but even if you can't afford one, consider who can help you around the house. This will be very important for when you have days that you feel sick or tired and don't feel like doing much, especially cleaning the bathroom. Think about what you might need such as someone to do the washing cooking or help with the housework.

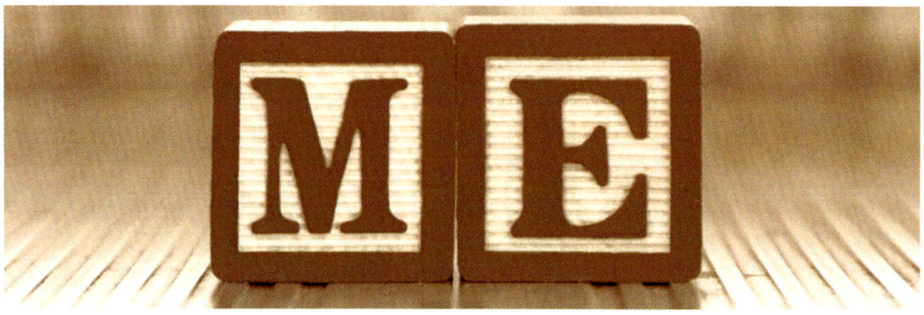

# SUPPORT

Receiving support when you have cancer is crucial for coping with the physical, emotional, and practical challenges that come with the diagnosis and treatment. It is hard to ask for support during this time especially if you have always been very independent but it is so important to know that you are not alone and have people who can help. Here are some ways to seek support:

1. **Lean on Loved Ones:** Reach out to family members, friends, and trusted individuals in your support network. Share your feelings, fears, and needs with them, and allow them to provide emotional support, companionship, and practical assistance.
2. **Join Support Groups:** Consider joining a cancer support group, either in person or online, where you can connect with others who are going through similar experiences. Sharing stories, advice, and encouragement with fellow cancer patients and survivors can provide validation, understanding, and a sense of community. You are going through something unique and finding others who know how you feel is going to make you feel less isolated.
3. **Seek Professional Support:** Consider working with a therapist, counsellor, or mental health professional who specializes in cancer-related issues. Professional support can help you navigate the emotional challenges of cancer, cope with anxiety and depression, and develop coping strategies for managing stress.
4. **Stay Informed:** Educate yourself about your cancer diagnosis, treatment options, and potential side effects. Ask questions and seek information from reliable sources, such as your healthcare providers, reputable websites, or cancer organizations. Understanding your condition can help you feel more empowered and involved in your care. Plus remember that there are new treatment developments every day.
5. **Communicate with Healthcare Providers:** Maintain open and honest communication with your healthcare team. Share your concerns, preferences, and treatment goals with them, and ask questions about your treatment plan, medications, and supportive care options. Your healthcare providers can offer guidance, support, and resources to help you manage your cancer journey effectively.
6. **Take Care of Yourself:** Prioritize self-care and well-being during your cancer treatment. Get plenty of rest, eat a healthy diet, engage in gentle exercise, and practice stress-reduction techniques such as meditation, deep breathing, or mindfulness. Taking care of yourself physically and emotionally can help you cope with the challenges of cancer more effectively.
7. **Explore Supportive Services:** Take advantage of supportive services and resources available to cancer patients, such as financial assistance programs, transportation services, complementary therapies (e.g., acupuncture, massage therapy), and integrative medicine programs. These services can help address practical needs and enhance your overall well-being during treatment.
8. **Stay Connected:** Stay connected with your support network and maintain social

connections with loved ones, even if it's through virtual means. Reach out to friends and family members for companionship, encouragement, and distraction from cancer-related stressors.

Remember that seeking support is a sign of strength, not weakness but we are all different and some people need more support than others. Don't hesitate to reach out for help when you need it, and remember that you're not alone in your cancer journey. With the right support and resources, you can navigate the challenges of cancer and may even emerge stronger and more resilient on the other side. The list of supports provided is just a starting place and will give you some ideas of where to start looking. Don't forget that you probably know of people who have gone through this. If you feel able reach out and ask questions, find out how they coped and what they did that worked. One friend of mine used to sit in a field with baby donkeys to make herself happy and I can honestly say that I thought it was the best idea I had ever heard of!

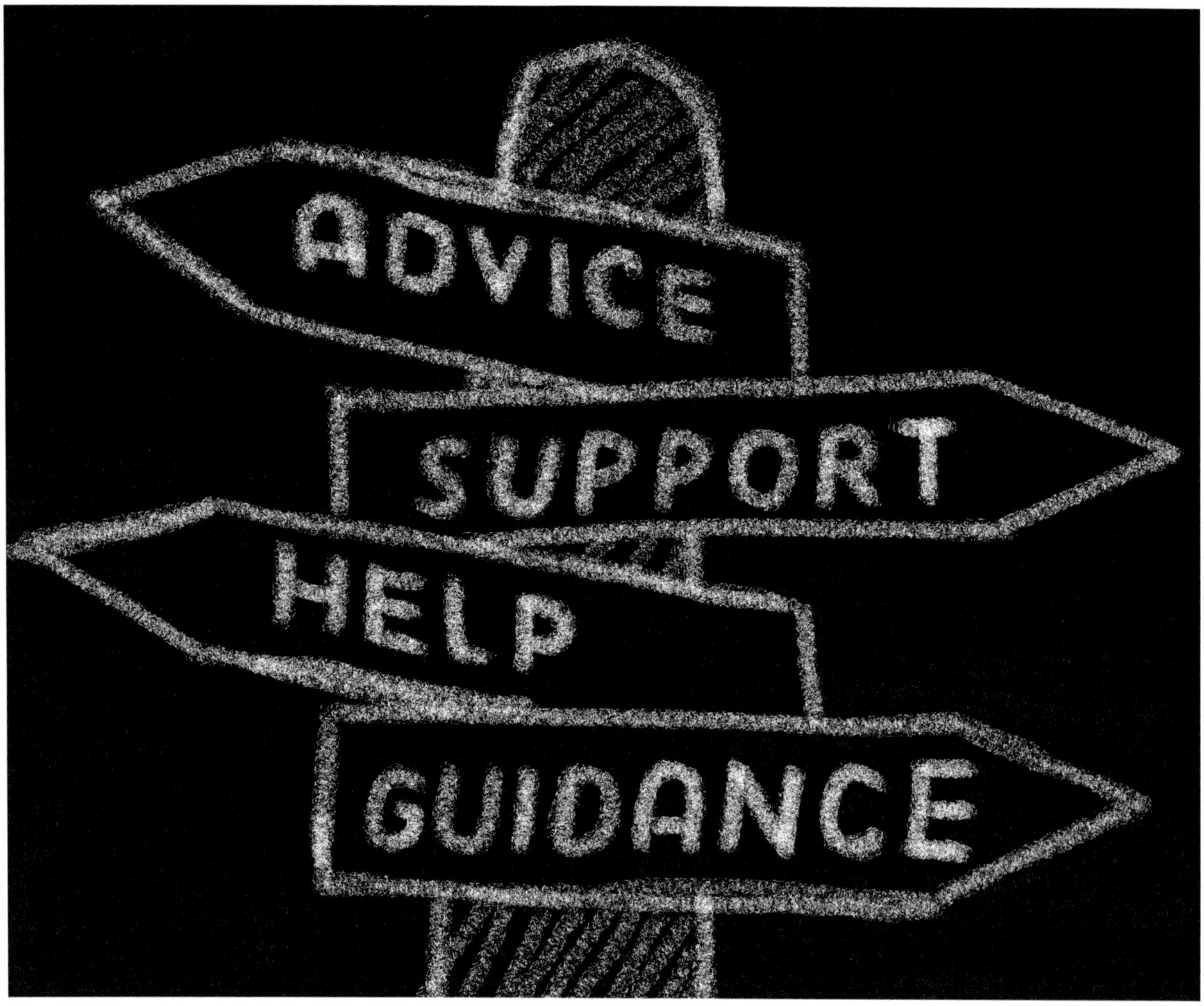

# HOW DO I TELL MY FAMILY?

Telling your loved ones, especially your partner and children, about a cancer diagnosis is a deeply personal and emotional conversation...lets face it it is horrible to be the one to deliver this news....or to receive it. One friend of mine blurted it out to her children then burst into tears. When the same friend told me of her diagnosis I yelled at her for nearly 20 minutes and told her it wasn't funny and why would she say this to me! I thought when I saw her call that she was ringing to tell me that she had bought shoes. It was the last thing I expected for her to tell me she had cancer. I was very much in shock and she took my reaction well considering how I had reacted. We laugh about it now but at the time it was not very funny and I never thought in my wildest dreams I would react in that way. There are lots of ways to tell people of your diagnosis and unfortunately there is no script. The people you love are possibly going to react in a number of different ways, shock, fear, and anger are emotions to be expected. Take you time and remember they love you and their job is going to be to support you. Here are some suggestions for how you might approach the conversation:

1. **Start with Love and Reassurance:** Begin the conversation by expressing your love and reassurance for your family. Let them know that what you're about to share is difficult but that you're all in this together as a family.
2. **Be Direct and Honest:** Use clear and straightforward language to convey your diagnosis. You might say something like, "I need to share some difficult news with you. I've been diagnosed with cancer."
3. **Provide Information:** Offer basic information about your diagnosis, such as the type of cancer, the stage (if known), and the treatment plan. Avoid overwhelming them with too many details initially, but let them know that you'll be sharing more information as it becomes available. When you know they will know. This is especially important for the key people in your life.
4. **Acknowledge Feelings:** Recognize that hearing news of a cancer diagnosis can be shocking and emotional. Allow your family members to express their feelings and reactions without judgment. Validate their emotions and reassure them that it's okay to feel scared, sad, or angry. Close family members may lash out and become very reactive due to shock. Don't take it personally (yes I realise what I am saying) but give them time to emotionally settle and then try to talk about it again. Unfortunately this is something that everyone will have to deal with in the family and it is not going away for a while and it won't just disappear if you ignore it.
5. **Encourage Questions:** Let your family know that you're available to answer any questions they may have about your diagnosis, treatment, or what to expect. Encourage open communication and let them know that no question is off-limits.
6. **Express Hope and Optimism:** While it's important to be honest about the challenges ahead, also express hope and optimism for the future. Let your family know that you're committed to fighting the cancer and that you have a supportive healthcare team and treatment plan in place.
7. **Emphasize Support:** Reassure your partner and children that you'll be leaning on

each other for support . Let them know that you're grateful for their love and support  and that you're in this together as a family

8. **Take Your Time:** Allow your family members time to process the news and react in their own way.  Give them time to freak out and then settle.  It is a shock and everyone is going to react differently.
9. **Seek Professional Help:** If you anticipate that the conversation may be particularly challenging or emotional, consider enlisting the support of a therapist, counsellor, or  social worker who can facilitate the conversation and provide additional support for your family members.

Remember that sharing news of a cancer diagnosis is a process, and it's okay to take it one step at a time when telling people you love. It is your news and you may need to take a few days to digest the information and consider how to tell people particularly if the family has had previous experience with cancer or illness.  A word of advice....if someone yells at you when you deliver the news it is only because they love you....and they are probably scared and in shock especially if they have never yelled at you before.

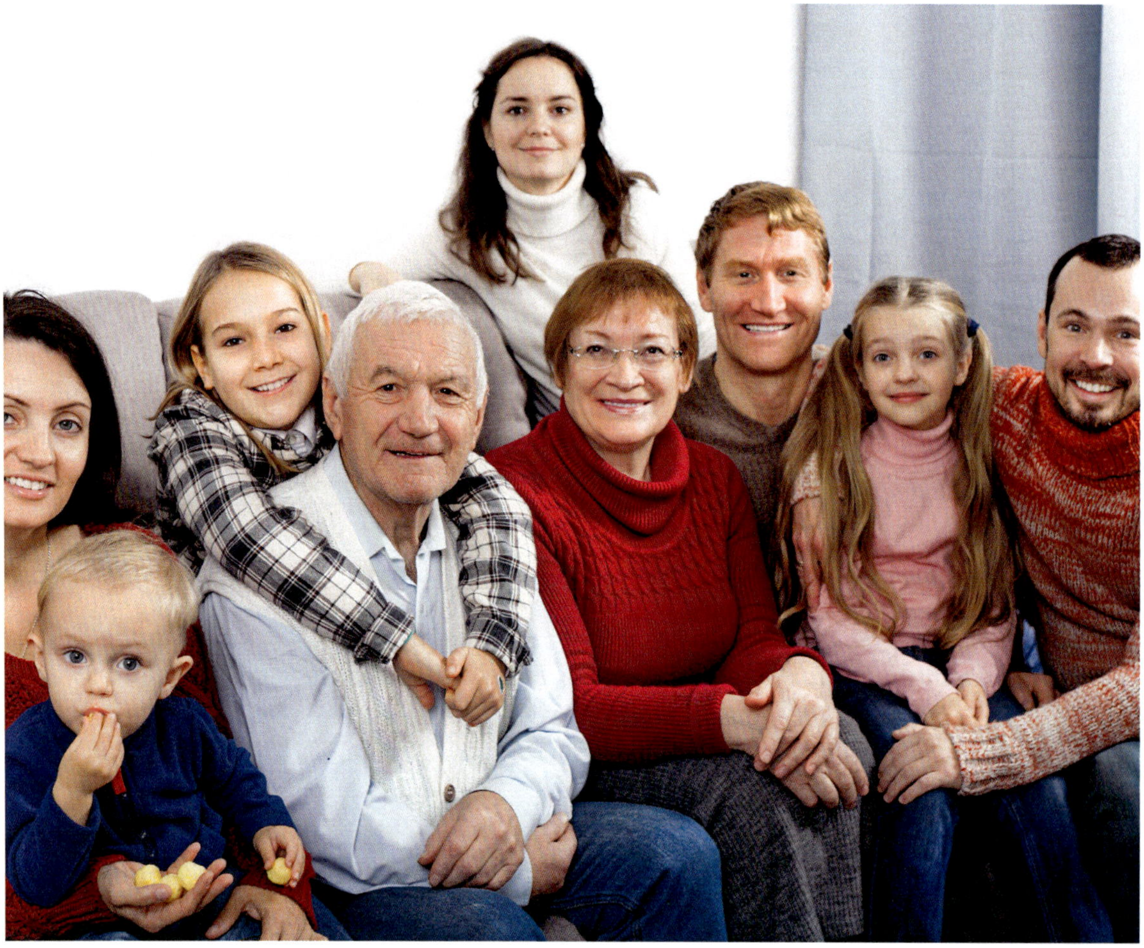

# WHAT DO I TELL PEOPLE?

Telling people that you have cancer is difficult but it is essential to communicate openly and honestly with those who are close to you. You can make a decision about the other people in your life and decide who to tell. After all everyone does not need to know everything and it is your information to share with whom you choose. Choose the friends who you want to tell and how much they need to know. Not everyone needs to know all the private details of your diagnosis especially if you find it difficult to speak about or if you are still wrapping your head around the diagnosis yourself. The important thing to remember is that this is your news and you have a right to be as public or private as you want to be. Here are some steps to consider when sharing your cancer diagnosis with others:

1. **Choose the Right Time and Place:** Select a comfortable and private setting where you can have a quiet conversation without interruptions as this will just make things much harder. Consider the emotional needs and preferences of both yourself and the person you're telling.
2. **Be Direct and Honest:** When sharing your diagnosis, be straightforward and honest about your condition. Use clear language to state the facts without minimizing or sugar coating the situation.
3. **Provide Information:** Offer information about your diagnosis, including the type of cancer, treatment plan, and prognosis, if this is known and your doctor has given you this information to make some decisions or time to prepare. Providing factual information can help reduce confusion and address the concerns of the person you are telling, which is understandable. Be clear about your treatment and other information concerning your case before you start this conversation as it might open up more questions than you know the answer to.
4. **Express Your Feelings (this is up to you):** Share your feelings and emotions about the diagnosis openly and authentically but only if you want to. It's okay to feel scared, sad, or overwhelmed, and expressing your emotions can help others understand what you're going through and how you feel about the situation.
5. **Ask for Support:** Let the person know how they can support you during this time. Whether it's offering practical assistance, emotional support, or simply being there to listen, communicating your needs can help others know how best to support you. Remember I have already suggested people can make you foods that you really want to eat or they may help with kids drop off or pick up from school. Play dates may also give you a break if you need a rest if you are not feeling well from medications.
6. **Give Them Space to React:** Allow the person time to process the news and react in their own way. Understand that they may experience a range of emotions, including shock, sadness, or concern. Also be ready for some people to not react at all. No one knows how they will react in the moment.

7. **Set Boundaries:** Establish boundaries around what you're comfortable sharing and how you want others to respond to your diagnosis. Let them know if there are topics or questions that are off-limits or if you prefer not to discuss certain aspects of your diagnosis.
8. **Offer Reassurance:** Assure the person that you're taking steps to address your diagnosis and that you have a supportive healthcare team and treatment plan in place. Offer reassurance that you're doing everything you can to manage your health and well-being. If they are struggling badly for whatever reason it might be that you have set off some issues that they might need to deal with. You are vulnerable yourself and there is going to be a limit to the amount of support you can offer. If needed suggest they seek additional support from a counsellor.
9. **Follow Up:** Well this might be a tricky one, you can choose to keep the lines of communication open but only if you want to. I would hope that your friends and close confidants check in on you and see how you are doing but not everyone knows how to react after this sort of information. The word cancer is also very scary and some people only hear the word and think the worst but there is plenty of evidence of people being diagnosed and doing treatment and living a long healthy life.

As I have already stated whom you tell and how much the people in your life "need to know" you tell is up too you. Not everyone may react the way you want them too but there will also (hopefully) be people who surpass your expectations and are the most surprising wonderful support for you and your family. These people are a gift.

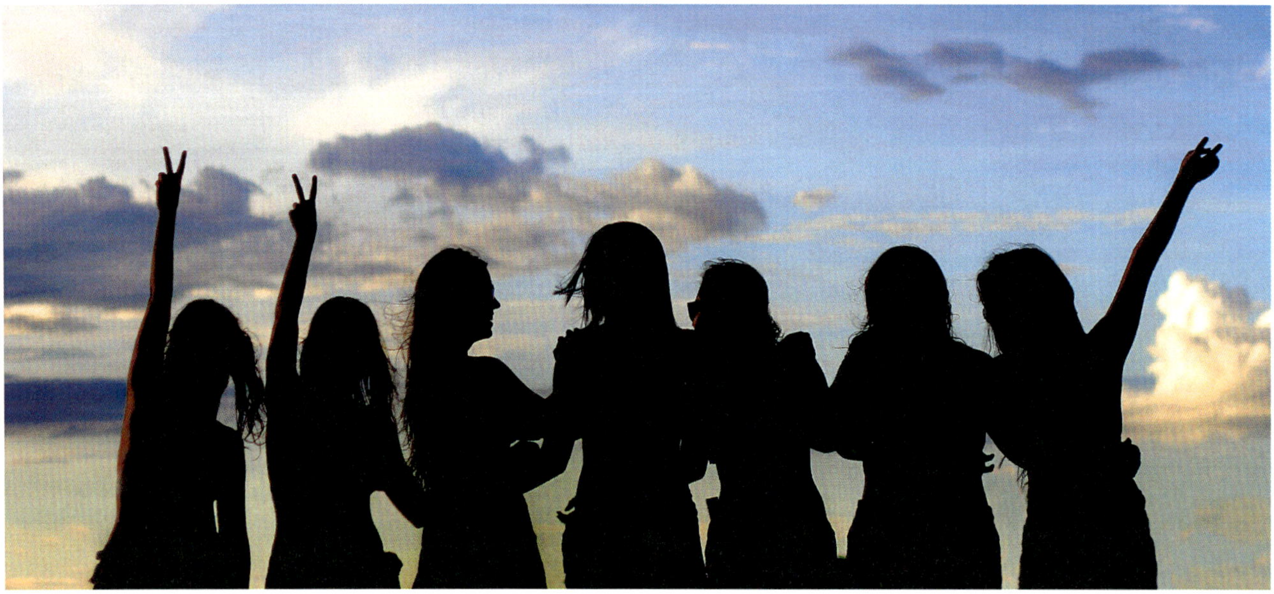

# HOW DO I TELL MY CHILDREN?

Telling your children about a cancer diagnosis can be one of the most challenging conversations you'll ever have....with anyone. I also don't think it matters if your children are young or old they are still going to be processing a lot of emotions as you are important to them and you are possibly going to need their help. They are also going to have a lot of fears about what is going to happen next especially if they have had little experience of cancer and the treatments that are involved. Here are some ways to approach this conversation:

1. **Choose the Right Time and Place:** Find a quiet, comfortable space where you can have a private conversation without distractions or interruptions. Consider a time when everyone is calm and relaxed, such as after a meal or during a weekend when you have uninterrupted time together. This will allow them to have your full attention while you try to explain your diagnosis.
2. **Start with Love and Reassurance:** Begin the conversation by expressing your love for your children and reassuring them that they're safe and loved. Let them know that what you're about to share is difficult but that you trust them to handle it together as a family.
3. **Use Clear and Age-Appropriate Language:** Tailor your language to the age and maturity level of your children. Use simple, age-appropriate language to explain what cancer is and how it affects your body. You might say something like the following to a younger child, "Mommy/Daddy has something called cancer, which is an illness that makes some cells in my body grow in a way they're not supposed to."
4. **Provide Information:** Offer basic information about your diagnosis, such as the type of cancer and the treatment plan. Avoid overwhelming them with too many details, but let them know what to expect in the coming days and weeks. Assure them that you have a team of doctors and nurses who are working hard to help you get better.
5. **Acknowledge Feelings:** Allow your children to express their feelings and reactions to the news. Encourage them to ask questions and share their thoughts, and validate their emotions by saying things like, "It's okay to feel scared or sad. I'm here to listen and help you understand."
6. **Offer Reassurance:** Reassure your children that they're not alone in this journey and that you'll be there to support each other every step of the way. Let them know that it's okay to ask questions and talk about their feelings, and that you're here to listen and provide comfort whenever they need it.
7. **Maintain Routine and Normalcy:** Try to maintain as much routine and normalcy as possible in your children's lives, despite the changes that cancer may bring. Stick to regular schedules for meals, bedtime, and activities, and make time for fun and laughter as a family such as a routine night to sit and watch a movie and spend time together as a family.
8. **Encourage Support:** Encourage your children to lean on other trusted adults, such as family members, friends, teachers, or counsellors, for additional support and

guidance. Let them know that it's okay to talk to someone else if they're feeling overwhelmed or need someone to listen. It might also be a good idea to organise a counsellor if they are struggling where they can talk about their fears and concerns about your diagnosis. If you have school aged children the school may have a counsellor already that you can contact and let them know your child needs some additional support.

9. **Stay Positive:** While it's important to be honest about the challenges ahead, also emphasize hope and optimism for the future. Let your children know that you're committed to fighting the cancer and that you have faith in your ability to overcome it together as a family.
10. **Follow Up:** Check in with your children regularly to see how they're coping with the news and offer ongoing support and reassurance. Be patient and understanding as they navigate their feelings and emotions, and remind them that you're here for them every step of the way.
11. **Be prepared:** Be prepared for them to react, lash out be angry and basically take out their emotions, fear and distress on you.....yes they know you are not well but they are children and they don't necessarily have the coping skills to be mature. Older children also may struggle and you can suggest additional supports and professional counselling to help them cope.

While this section might feel like it is aimed at younger children in my experience no one ever reacts well when a parent they love tells them they are ill. It makes sense to apply the same strategies to children of all ages...even the older ones when telling them of your diagnosis.

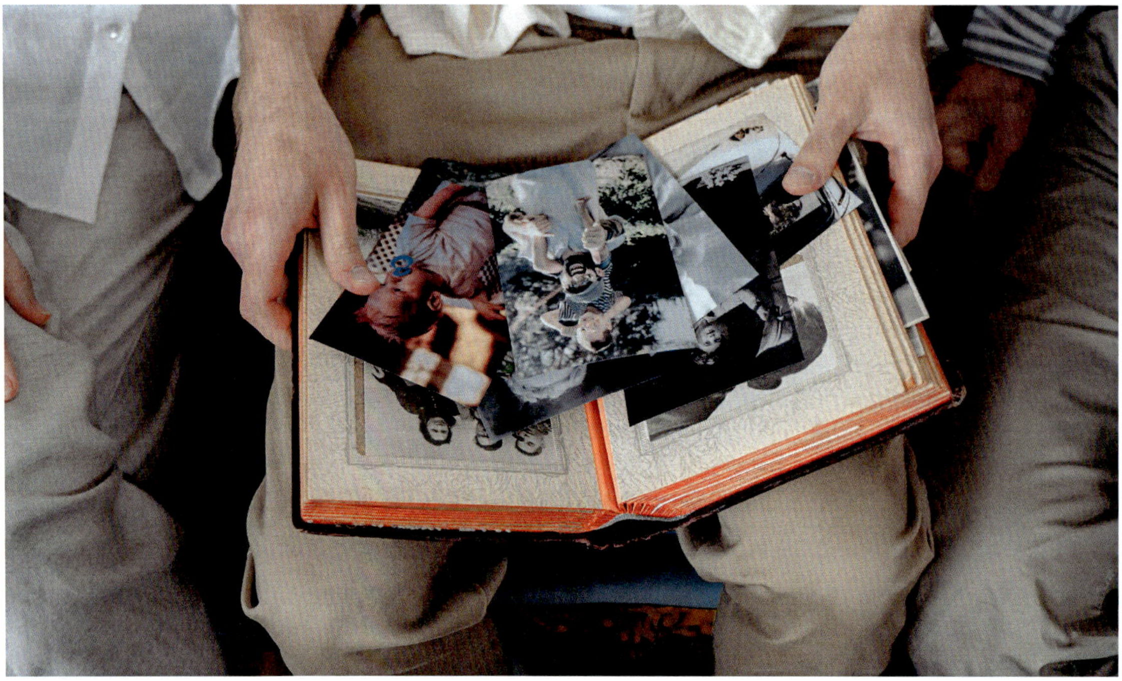

# SUPPORT CREW!

Emotional support is so important and people will want to help you....let them! Put your own nerves and issues to one side and let people who love and want to support you, take care of you. There will be people that you pull in very close who will provide love and support and be there every step of the way and there will be others who will be nervous and be a bit unsure of what to do. Either way people are surprising (especially who turns up to help and in what ways)! Given the situation think about what you might need and who are going to be the best people to give it to you....even if what you need is a laugh.

1. **Who are my crew?:** These are your people and there may only be a few of them or you might be lucky and have lots. Your crew may only include your partner or best friend. You may also have family or parents who are able to help. Whoever they are write their names down on the next page. These are the people who are really going to be in your corner. These people are going to be the ones you will have to have the difficult conversations with and they are the ones you call in your darkest moments for support.
2. **Who will you be able to rely on and can they really help?:** Think about what you may need from people. Do you need help getting to hospital or appointments? Do you need people to help you with getting the kids to sports, or help you with your pets. Make a list of what you are going to need and who can help.
3. **Be realistic:** Human beings are funny creatures and they can react in some funny ways when you tell them you are ill. They either can't cope because they feel unsure of what to do or say or they are unable to cope with the severity of your diagnosis as they only think the worst! These people still love you but they are not going to give you what you need right now. Also there are others who let you down and although you thought you could rely on them in the past, in reality they are not who you thought they were. While it might be upsetting if someone lets you down take time and look at who you do have in your corner and lean on these people for support.
4. **Be surprised!:** While there are some people who will let you down you may also find support where you least expected it....During a time like this some surprising people come out of the woodwork and really step up to help you.......Embrace these people and pull them close you are going to need them.
5. **Meet up:** It might be a good idea for the support crew to meet and get to know each other. This way they can help you and organise things that you might need. Plus they may also need to support each other while you are ill, they love you and they are going to find all of the changes and stages you are about to go though very difficult. This way they can support each other as well as you.
6. **Be careful who you choose:** Pick people who are going to be positive and have a laugh with you in some dark moments....totally gold! You don't want people around you who are dramatic and have their own issues to deal with or will make it about them. Right now it is all about you! I have one friend who said the most important thing was that her friends just treated her as normal and still had a laugh.

## MY GANG

## WHO CAN DO WHAT?

# SUPPORT PARTNER!

Emotional support is so important and here are some rules if you are a partner or friend. Remember this will not be over in 5 minutes but you are the support crew for a marathon runner.......and whether you are at the start, middle, or end of someone's treatment you are an essential part of the process. Don't promise help and then not give it....people are going to rely on you.  If you are going to be part of the crew then only commit to what you can give.

1. **Be There**: Simply being present and available to listen can provide immense comfort to someone with cancer. Let them know that you're there for them and willing to offer support in whatever way they need.
2. **Educate Yourself:** Take the time to learn about your loved one's type of cancer, treatment options, and potential side effects. Be mindful of not giving advice about alternate therapies or "magical cures"  as they are already struggling with options for treatment and making lots of decisions.  Do not be a Dr Google advice giver....be a support.
3. **Offer Practical Help:** Offer to assist with daily tasks such as cooking, cleaning, grocery shopping, or running errands. Even small gestures can make a big difference and alleviate some of the practical burdens they may be facing.
4. **Provide Emotional Support:** Be empathetic, compassionate, and understanding. Allow your loved one to express their feelings and emotions without judgment. Offer a listening ear, a shoulder to lean on, or a comforting presence when needed.
5. **Respect Their Wishes:** Respect your loved one's autonomy and preferences regarding their treatment, care, and decisions. Offer support and guidance without imposing your own opinions or agendas, unless specifically asked and remember you are not their treating physician.
6. **Be Flexible:** Understand that your loved one's needs and preferences may change throughout their cancer journey. Be flexible and adaptable in your support, and be willing to adjust your approach based on their evolving needs.
7. **Offer Distractions:** Help them find moments of joy and distraction from their cancer diagnosis by engaging in activities they enjoy, such as watching movies, going for walks, or pursuing hobbies together. My friend and I looked at shoe websites and talked about renovations as distractions.....do what works!
8. **Provide Practical Resources:** Help your loved one access practical help such as support groups, counselling, financial assistance programs, or transportation services.
9. **Respect Privacy:** Respect your loved one's privacy and boundaries regarding their cancer diagnosis. Avoid sharing personal information or updates about their health without their consent, it is their news to tell.
10. **Take Care of Yourself:** Supporting someone with cancer can be emotionally and physically exhausting. It's essential to maintain your own well-being so that you can continue to be a source of strength and support for your loved one.
11. **Treatment:** Treat them as normally as you can......they are still the same person!

# I HAVE A DEPENDENT?

There are a few things to consider if you have a someone who is dependant upon you. In this situation you may be elderly or your partner or family member is dependant upon you for their own needs and wellbeing. You may need to consider who can help you and what sort of support your partner or family member may require. Please consider these things as early as you can as it may take some time to organise some aspects of care. Here are some things to consider:

**Practical Supports:**

1. **Home Health Aides and Professional Caregivers:**
   - Hiring a professional caregiver or home health aide can provide assistance with daily activities, medical care, and companionship for your dependent family member.
   - These professionals can help with tasks such as bathing, dressing, medication management, and mobility assistance.
   - Also consider if your dependant are part of the NDIS. Ask if a plan review can be organised so that additional supports can be implemented.
2. **Respite Care:**
   - Respite care offers temporary relief for primary caregivers by providing short-term care for the dependent family member.
   - Respite care services can be arranged through home care agencies, nursing homes, or community organizations. You might need this when you are in hospital or you need a rest from your family member during treatment.
3. **Adult Day Care Centres:**
   - These centres provide a safe and supportive environment for special needs adults during the day, offering activities, meals, and medical care.
   - This option allows you to focus on your treatment and recovery while ensuring your family member is well cared for.
4. **Community Resources and Support Services:**
   - Local community organizations, churches, and social services often offer support programs for families dealing with illness.
   - Look for meal delivery services, transportation assistance, and volunteer programs that can help with daily tasks.

**Emotional and Psychological Supports:**

1. **Counselling and Therapy:**
   - Individual or family counselling can provide emotional support, help manage stress, and improve coping strategies for both you and your dependent family member. This might be specialised help if your family member has limited understanding or a disability.
   - Therapists can offer guidance on how to communicate effectively and address the emotional challenges of dealing with cancer. They can help you to address the fears your family member might be feeling.

2. **Support Groups:**
    - Joining a support group for cancer patients and caregivers can provide a sense of community, shared experiences, and practical advice.
    - It might be worth checking out the groups that might be attached to the hospital or on Facebook.
3. **Mental Health Services:**
    - If your dependent family member has mental health needs, ensure they have access to appropriate mental health services, such as therapy or psychiatric care. You might need to seek extra support when you are going through treatment.
    - Consider telehealth options for convenience and continuity of care.

**Financial and Logistical Supports:**

1. **Financial Assistance Programs:**
    - Explore financial assistance programs for cancer patients, which can help cover treatment costs, transportation, and caregiving expenses.
    - Organizations like the the Cancer Council offer resources.
2. **Legal and Advocacy Services:**
    - Consult with a social worker or legal advocate to understand your rights and access services like disability benefits, insurance coverage, and caregiver support programs.
    - These professionals can also help with advance care planning and legal documentation.
3. **Family and Friends:**
    - Reach out to family and friends for help with caregiving duties, household chores, and emotional support.
    - Don't hesitate to ask for specific assistance, such as driving to appointments, preparing meals, or spending time with your dependent family member.

**Self-Care and Personal Well-Being:**

1. **Prioritize Your Health:**
    - Make sure to follow your treatment plan, attend medical appointments, and take medications as prescribed. While it is tempting with other pressures building up to ignore your treatment...don't.
    - Practice self-care by getting enough rest, eating a balanced diet, and engaging in relaxation techniques like meditation or gentle exercise.
2. **Set Boundaries:**
    - Recognize your limits and set boundaries to avoid burnout. Communicate your needs clearly to family members and caregivers. Ask for help when needed.
    - Delegate tasks whenever possible and accept help when offered.
3. **Create a Care Plan:**
    - Develop a comprehensive care plan that outlines the responsibilities and needs of both you and your dependent family member. This is so important.
    - Include contact information for healthcare providers, emergency plans, and a schedule for caregiving duties.

By utilizing these strategies and resources, you can better manage the care of your dependent family member while focusing on your own health and well-being during cancer treatment. Remember that seeking support and delegating tasks are crucial steps in maintaining a balance and ensuring both you and your loved one receive the care you need.

**NOTES**

# SUPPORT FOR YOU IN HOSPITAL!

While you are in hospital you may need some people to come and distract you as you will probably get bored and crave company. You might also need some practical help such as someone to bring you socks or extra clothes.

1. **Emotional Support:** Ask your close friends and family to come and visit. Having someone to talk to, express your feelings, fears, and worries can be incredibly comforting. It's important to have someone who listens without judgment and provides empathy and understanding. In addition, you may want people to come and visit because hospital can be a very confusing, boring place and full of people who are constantly taking your temperature and asking if you want a cup of tea every 5 minutes. A familiar face is a welcome relief!
2. **Advocacy:** Sometimes navigating the healthcare system can be overwhelming, especially when dealing with a serious illness like cancer. Having someone who can advocate for you, ask questions, and ensure you receive the care you need is invaluable. Not everyone knows what questions to ask or has medical professionals in the family. It can be nice to feel less alone and have someone else to remember the important bits. Also consider if you want a close friend to also be able to access your condition in hospital and be on the contact list.
3. **Provide Comfort Items:** Bring comfort items from home to help the you feel more comfortable during your hospital stay. A favourite blanket, pillow, clothing, books, music, or other personal items that provide comfort and familiarity. Fluffy socks also help as your feet can get really cold. **Remember no flowers on a cancer ward! I didn't know that either until I started to work on this book!!!** Remember to tell people who want to visit to wear a mask as you might be immunocompromised!
4. **Companionship:** Hospital stays can be lonely, especially when you're dealing with a serious illness. Having someone to keep you company, offer distractions, or simply sit with you can provide comfort and companionship during difficult times is wonderful. I cannot say it enough....**pick the right people** to support you and those who can handle your treatment. You need people who are going to be in your corner and also treat you the same as they did before. It will help you to feel more normal in the most abnormal surreal experience that is cancer diagnosis and treatment.
5. **Information and Education**: It's essential to understand your diagnosis, treatment options, and what to expect during your hospital stay. Having someone who can help you gather information, ask questions, and understand medical jargon can empower you to make informed decisions about your care.
6. **Support from Healthcare Professionals:** In addition to support from loved ones, it is crucial to have a supportive healthcare team that provides compassionate care, addresses your concerns, and involves you in your treatment decisions. In reality you will not have a lot of control as your treatment regime is tailored to your cancer type but you do want to feel consulted and that you are not just a number.

7. **Encouragement and Motivation:** Dealing with cancer can be exhausting, both physically and emotionally. Having someone who provides encouragement, motivation, and positivity can help you stay strong and hopeful during your hospitalization. This is so important and you need people about who are going to be upbeat and not weep and wail when it is the last thing you need....I have asked my friends who have gone through treatment what it is I can do (as I wasn't sure and although I'm a psychologist I felt helpless) and rather than giving them what I thought they wanted I asked what they wanted! They both said "treat me the same as always" and "make me laugh". So that's what I did! Humour can sometimes be found in some very dark places.
8. **Medication:** Some of the medication you might get in hospital might make you a bit odd. Warn family members. One friend made the nurses cry and was put in a room by herself which was for storage and then she called me constantly because she was bored!!! I was at work and couldn't answer....she got increasingly more demanding until I did answer and she wanted to know if I had seen the photos of her in the storage room and did I know she made a nurse cry....I couldn't stop laughing and told her to behave. My other friend talked non stop.....without drawing breath and even answered her own questions......see what I mean.....you can always find something to laugh about.

You won't be in hospital all the time during your treatment but it helps to have an idea of what to expect. Sometimes this is the first time someone has been in hospital and hospitals can be a very daunting place especially when you feel vulnerable. Hospitals are a weird melting pot of noises and weird smells, people everywhere and lots of noise. Ironically there is nothing quiet about a hospital.

# ADVOCACY

Advocating for your medical treatment is crucial to ensure you receive the care that aligns with your needs and preferences while still targeting your cancer. Here are some strategies to think about:

**Educate Yourself**

1. **Understand Your Condition:** Learn about your illness, treatment options, potential side effects, and prognosis. Reliable sources include medical websites, support groups, and literature provided by healthcare professionals.
2. **Know Your Rights:** Familiarize yourself with patient rights, including informed consent, the right to refuse treatment, and privacy protections under laws like HIPAA in the U.S. or the 1988 Privacy Act in Australia which relate to Private Health Information.

**Communication Strategies**

1. **Prepare for Appointments:** Write down questions and concerns before your medical appointments. Bring a list of symptoms, medications, and any other relevant information. Yes you might feel a bit unpopular with the doctor if they have a waiting room full of people, but they work for you and you have a right to ask questions. It is your body and a lot is going on.
2. **Ask Questions:** Don't hesitate to ask for clarification on anything you don't understand. Use the "teach-back" method where you repeat back what the doctor has told you to ensure that you are understanding the information correctly.
3. **Be Honest and Open:** Share all relevant information about your symptoms, lifestyle, and concerns. This helps your doctor make the best recommendations for your treatment.
4. **Be respectful:** The doctor is working hard for you and they have years of experience in what they are doing. However, if you feel something is "not right" ask, and question. Think about what you would do if it was your child or a loved one who was in the same position. If you wouldn't accept it for your child why is it good enough for you? This perspective may help you to find the right answer when you are concerned.

**Building a Support Team**

1. **Involve a Support Person:** Bring a trusted friend or family member to appointments to help listen, take notes, and ask questions. One friend of mine only heard half the information which was a bit problematic as she told everyone she was cured when she wasn't.......She just got excited and jumped the gun a bit.....but this highlights how important a support person in appointments can be.
2. **Collaborate with Your Healthcare Team:** View your relationship with your healthcare providers as a partnership. Respect their expertise, but also make sure they respect your preferences and values. I'm going to say it...While crystals and new age treatments are wonderful they are not necessarily going to cure you so take

medical advice seriously and the team know more than Google! Alternative treatments can support your recovery but lets face it, you are going to need the good drugs and treatments to get through this. I will say though that everyone I know who has had cancer I am the first in line to buy them crystals (curated to their type of cancer) and then tell them to get the Chemo. People are vulnerable at this time and everyone wants the miracle cure.  I wish there was one but there isn't.

**Decision-Making Strategies**

1. **Weigh the Options:** When presented with treatment options, consider the risks, benefits, and how they align with your goals and values.
2. **Seek Second Opinions:** If unsure about a diagnosis or treatment plan, don't hesitate to get a second opinion from another healthcare professional.
3. **Advance Directives:** Consider creating advance directives, such as a living will and durable power of attorney for healthcare, to outline your wishes in case you become unable to communicate them.

**Practical Steps**

1. **Document Everything:** Keep a personal health record with all your medical information, including test results, treatment plans, and communications with healthcare providers. There is space at the back of this book for this reason.
2. **Use Technology:** Utilize patient portals to access your medical records, communicate with your healthcare team, and stay informed about your health status.
3. **Stay Organized:** Use a calendar to keep track of appointments, medication schedules, and important health-related events.

**Advocacy Skills**

1. **Be Assertive:** Politely but firmly communicate your needs and preferences. Practice assertiveness techniques if necessary.
2. **Know When to Escalate:** If you feel your concerns are not being addressed, know how to escalate the issue. This might involve speaking to a patient advocate, contacting the hospital administration, or seeking legal advice. Check in with a close friend/family member to make sure that you are being reasonable and if they say you are not just wait before firing off that angry email. It might be the medication talking. A good therapist can come in handy at this point.
3. **Stay Informed:** Keep up with the latest developments in your condition and treatments. Subscribing to medical journals, joining support groups, or following relevant organizations can be beneficial.

**Emotional and Psychological Support**

1. **Seek Emotional Support:** Engage with support groups, counsellors, or therapists to help cope with the emotional aspects of advocating for your treatment.
2. **Mind-Body Practices:** Techniques such as mindfulness, meditation, and yoga can help reduce stress and improve your overall well-being.

**Utilizing Resources**

1. **Patient Advocacy Services:** Many hospitals and healthcare systems have patient advocates who can assist you in navigating the healthcare system and resolving issues.
2. **Legal Aid:** If you face discrimination or your rights are violated, legal aid services can provide assistance and support.

By being proactive, informed, and assertive, you can effectively advocate for your medical treatment and ensure that your healthcare needs are met in a way that aligns with your personal values and preferences. However, be mindful that your team is there to work for you and it is ok to question things it is your body after all.

# WHEN THINGS ARE NOT GOOD

Advocating for yourself when cancer treatment is **not** going well can be challenging but is essential to ensure you receive the best care possible. Here are some strategies to help you advocate effectively:

**Educate Yourself**

1. **Understand Your Condition:** Familiarize yourself with the specifics of your cancer type, stage, and standard treatment protocols. Reliable sources include cancer organizations, medical journals, and healthcare providers.
2. **Know the Alternatives:** Research alternative treatments or clinical trials that may be available for your type of cancer.

**Communication Strategies**

1. **Be Honest and Direct:** Clearly communicate your symptoms, side effects, and concerns to your healthcare team. Don't downplay what you are experiencing.
2. **Ask Questions:** Don't hesitate to ask your doctors to explain complex medical terms or treatment plans in a way you can understand. Ask about the goals of your current treatment, potential side effects, and what other options might be available.
3. **Request Detailed Explanations:** When treatments are not working, ask your oncologist to explain why and discuss potential next steps. Understanding the rationale behind decisions can help you make informed choices.

**Building a Support Team**

1. **Bring an Advocate:** Have a trusted friend or family member accompany you to appointments to help take notes, ask questions, and provide emotional support. Very important...remember my friend who jumped the gun and thought she was cured.....also a trusted friend can validate if you have concerns or tell you if you are being unreasonable.
2. **Collaborate with Your Healthcare Team:** Build a cooperative relationship with your healthcare providers, ensuring they see you as an active participant in your care. There is no I in Team....an oldie but a goodie. The relationship is a collaboration and needs to work for you to optimise outcomes.

**Decision-Making Strategies**

1. **Seek Second Opinions:** If you are not satisfied with your current treatment plan, seek a second opinion from another oncologist or a cancer centre that specializes in your type of cancer. You could also talk to your GP for advice.
2. **Explore Clinical Trials:** Investigate whether there are clinical trials available that might be suitable for your condition. Your oncologist or a research nurse can help you find and evaluate clinical trials.
3. **Consider Palliative Care:** Palliative care focuses on improving quality of life and managing symptoms. It can be used alongside curative treatments or as part of a transition to end-of-life care.

**Practical Steps**

1. **Document Your Journey:** Keep a detailed record of your symptoms, treatments, side effects, and any communications with your healthcare team. This information can be invaluable during appointments and when seeking second opinions.
2. **Utilize Patient Portals:** Use online patient portals to access your medical records, communicate with your healthcare team, and stay informed about your treatment progress.

**Advocacy Skills**

1. **Be Assertive:** Politely but firmly advocate for your needs and preferences. Practice assertiveness techniques if necessary.
2. **Escalate When Necessary:** If your concerns are not being addressed, don't hesitate to escalate the issue. This could involve speaking to a patient advocate, contacting the hospital administration, or seeking legal advice if your rights are being infringed upon.
3. **Stay Informed:** Continuously educate yourself about your condition and treatment options. Being well-informed empowers you to make better decisions.

**Emotional and Psychological Support**

1. **Seek Emotional Support:** Engage with support groups, counsellors, or therapists to help cope with the emotional toll of cancer treatment.
2. **Mind-Body Practices:** Techniques such as mindfulness, meditation, and yoga can help manage stress and improve your overall well-being. After all do what works and there is lots of evidence to suggest that adjunct therapies can help you to cope.

**Utilizing Resources**

1. **Patient Advocacy Services:** Many hospitals and cancer treatment centres have patient advocates who can assist you in navigating the healthcare system and resolving issues.
2. **Legal Aid:** If you face discrimination or your rights are violated, legal aid services can provide assistance and support.

**Consider Quality of Life**

1. **Reassess Goals:** Regularly reassess your treatment goals with your healthcare team. Sometimes, the focus might shift from curative treatment to managing symptoms and maintaining quality of life.
2. **Palliative Care Consultation:** Even if you are still pursuing active treatment, a palliative care consultation can provide additional support in managing symptoms and improving quality of life. We talk about this more in the sealed section!

Advocating for yourself requires persistence, knowledge, and sometimes the courage to push for what you believe is best for your health and well-being.

# I'M SCARED

It is a huge thing to be given a cancer diagnosis and it is normal for you to be worried/scared/frightened and generally terrified. Frankly I would be slightly surprised if you were not expressing some concerns and fears. On the next few pages there is some information about how your body and brain might be responding to your diagnosis. It is **normal** to feel anxious and worried and for you to have good and bad days. Anxiety and panic is also normal as there are lots of unknowns. However, if you understand how your body and brain are reacting when you feel worried you can use strategies to help you manage your symptoms so that you can focus on what you need to focus on which is treatment and getting well.

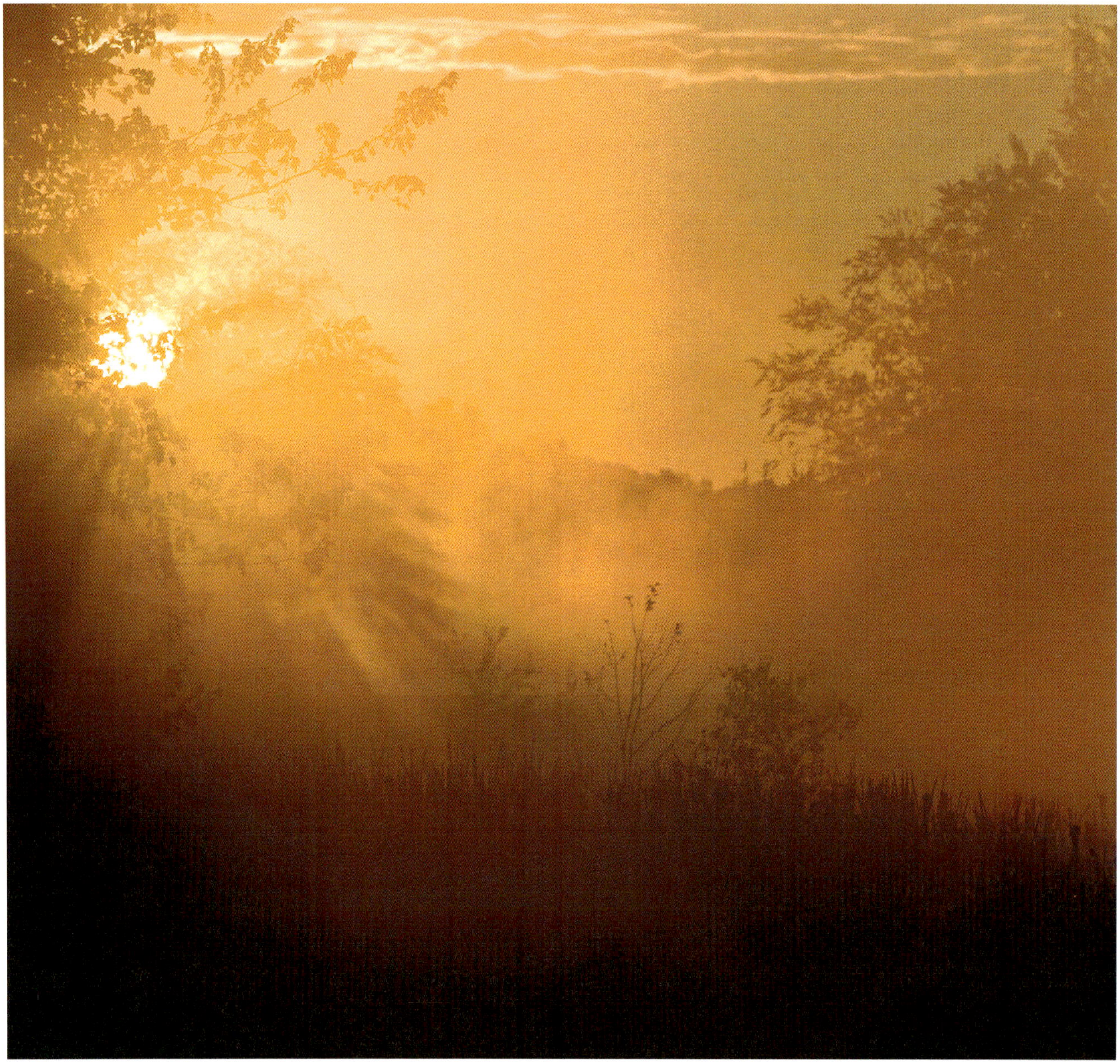

# MEDICAL TRAUMA

Medical trauma refers to the psychological and emotional distress experienced as a result of medical treatment or procedures. It can occur in various healthcare settings, including hospitals, clinics, and doctor's offices, and can affect patients of all ages. Here are some key points about medical trauma:

1. **Types of Medical Trauma:** Medical trauma can result from a variety of experiences, including invasive procedures, surgeries, emergency medical interventions, hospitalization, diagnosis of serious or life-threatening conditions (such as cancer), complications during treatment, adverse reactions to medication, and negative interactions with healthcare providers.
2. **Symptoms:** Symptoms of medical trauma can vary widely and may include anxiety, depression, panic attacks, nightmares, flashbacks of medical experiences, avoidance of medical settings or procedures, hypervigilance regarding health, difficulty trusting healthcare providers, and challenges with coping or adapting to medical conditions. You can also experience triggers to reminders of your treatment that appear even after you have finished your treatment. For example, you may suddenly become distressed or feel sick if you drink a cordial you drank while undergoing treatment in hospital. These negative associations are often underestimated but they are very debilitating when they suddenly turn up and you were not expecting them to impact you. After all Cordial can seem pretty harmless....If you then encounter it in a social setting....you may get triggered by the association and suffer flashbacks and distress as a result.
3. **Risk Factors:** Certain factors may increase the risk of experiencing medical trauma, including a history of trauma or mental health disorders, previous negative medical experiences, sensitivity to pain or medical procedures, lack of support or communication from healthcare providers, and feelings of powerlessness or lack of control over medical decisions.
4. **Impact:** Medical trauma can have significant consequences for patients' physical and emotional well-being, as well as their healthcare experiences and outcomes. It may interfere with treatment adherence, lead to avoidance of necessary medical care, contribute to increased healthcare utilization, and negatively affect overall quality of life.
5. **Treatment:** Addressing medical trauma often requires a multifaceted approach that prioritizes patient-centred care, trauma-informed practices, and psychological support. This may include providing information and education about medical procedures, fostering open communication and collaboration between patients and healthcare providers, offering emotional support and validation of patients' experiences, and utilizing trauma-focused therapies (such as cognitive-behavioural therapy or eye movement desensitization and reprocessing) to process and heal from traumatic experiences.

Recognizing and addressing medical trauma is essential for promoting compassionate and patient-centred healthcare that prioritizes the psychological well-being and dignity of all individuals receiving medical treatment. Some people can develop trauma symptoms as a result of their diagnosis or treatment. They can want to avoid people and places that might "trigger" those fear responses. However, people who develop a fear based response to medical procedures and places may need to be able to overcome these issues to ensure that their treatment and recovery is not compromised. In this case it is important for you to know that fear is normal and in fact it can help motivate you to seek treatment. It is when the fear is so overwhelming that you are unable to move, act, or do what you need to do....then we have a problem and we need to do something about it.

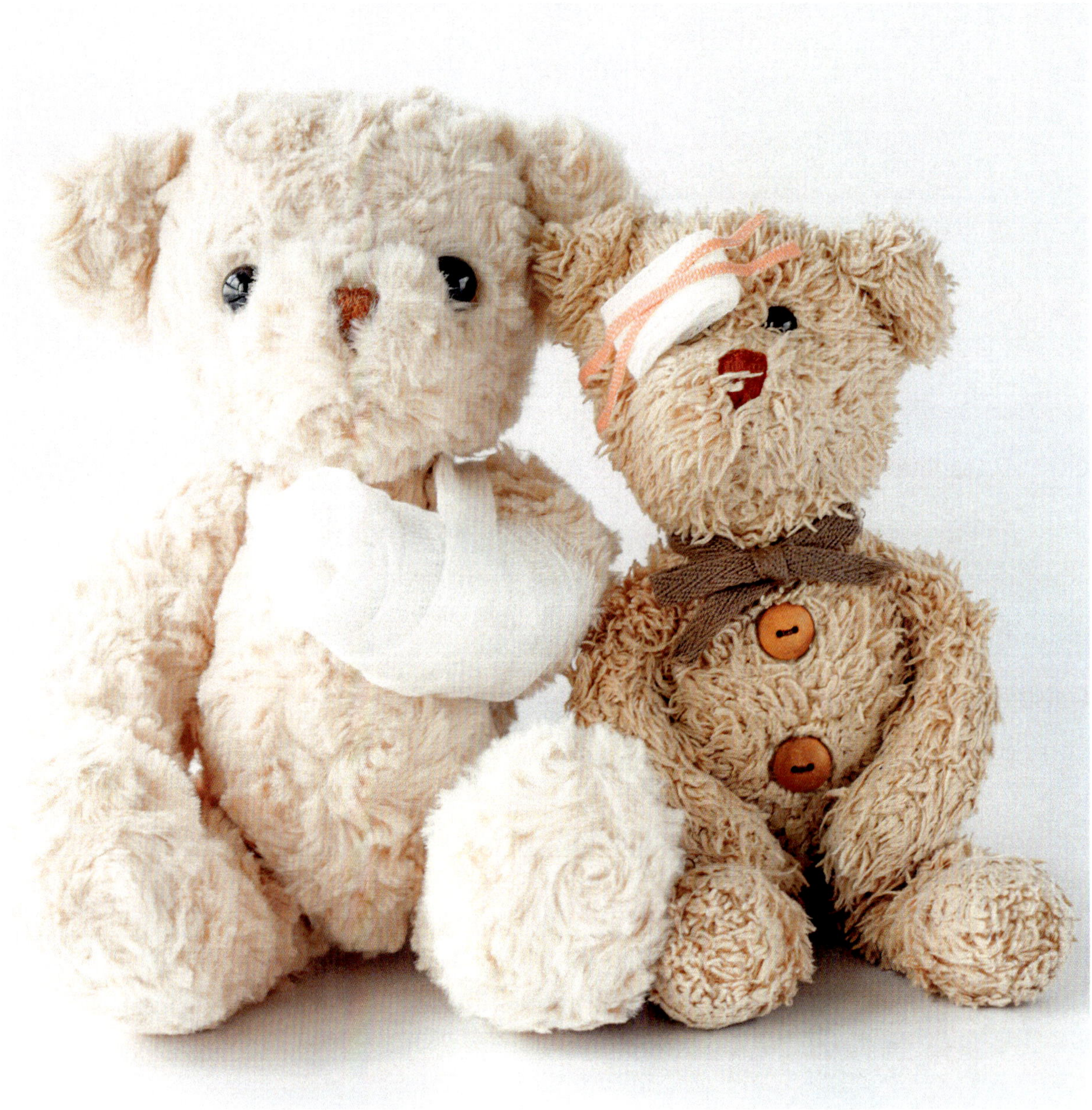

# SYMPTOMS OF TRAUMA

Post-traumatic stress disorder (PTSD) can occur in individuals who have experienced or witnessed a traumatic event, and this can include a cancer diagnosis and treatment. While cancer is not often associated with trauma the the emotional and psychological impact of this diagnosis can be profound and may lead to PTSD in some cases. Here are some ways in which cancer can contribute to PTSD:

1. **Traumatic Diagnosis:** Being diagnosed with cancer can be a traumatic event in itself. It can shatter one's sense of safety and security and lead to feelings of fear, anxiety, and uncertainty about the future. You might feel really angry that your "body has betrayed you" and it is not doing what you "expected". This can make you feel vulnerable and frightened.
2. **Treatment Trauma:** Cancer treatments such as chemotherapy, radiation therapy, and surgery can be physically and emotionally taxing. There is all of the medical tests which can be invasive and it seems like everyone is talking about you and to you in a different language. There are a series of doctors who talk to you about things that make no sense that are happening in your body in medical speak and jargon that sounds bizarre. Also once you are in hospital to start treatment there is a well meaning nurse every 5 minutes (or it feels like it) taking your blood pressure, temperature, giving you an injection, putting in a port (for medications) or hooking you up to something weird that is a weird colour that is supposed to make you feel better. The side effects, pain, and discomfort associated with these treatments not to mention losing your hair (but not always) can be traumatic experiences for many patients.
3. **Fear of Recurrence:** Even after successful treatment, many cancer survivors live with a fear of the cancer returning. This constant fear and worry about recurrence can be emotionally distressing and can contribute to symptoms of PTSD. This is very normal and it is expected that you would have anxiety about fear of recurrence. We will go into this in more detail in a later section of this book. We will also help you to find some ways to cope with your "fear thinking".
4. **Loss and Grief:** Cancer often involves significant losses, including loss of physical health, loss of independence, and loss of roles and identity. Dealing with these losses can trigger feelings of grief and contribute to PTSD symptoms. We will also discuss this in more detail later in the book.
5. **Isolation and Social Support:** Cancer diagnosis and treatment can lead to social isolation and strained relationships with friends and family. Feeling isolated and lacking social support can exacerbate feelings of trauma and distress.

It's important for individuals who have been diagnosed with cancer to receive comprehensive support, including psychological support, to address the emotional and psychological impact of the disease. This may involve therapy, support groups, medication, and other interventions aimed at managing symptoms of PTSD and improving overall well-being.

# TRAUMATIC DIAGNOSIS

Post-traumatic stress disorder (PTSD) is a mental health condition that can develop after experiencing or witnessing a traumatic event. Traumatic events can include but are not limited to military combat, natural disasters, sexual or physical assault, serious accidents, or acts of terrorism the one we don't often talk about is medical trauma or trauma associated with a life threatening illness or diagnosis. The word cancer is terrifying for most people. PTSD is characterized by a range of symptoms that persist beyond the initial traumatic experience and significantly impact daily functioning. There are several key aspects to PTSD:

1. **Symptoms:**
   - **Intrusive Thoughts:** Recurrent and distressing memories, flashbacks, or nightmares related to the traumatic event.
   - **Avoidance:** Avoiding reminders, thoughts, or situations associated with the trauma.
   - **Negative Mood and Thoughts:** Persistent negative emotions, feelings of detachment, loss of interest in previously enjoyed activities, and distorted beliefs about oneself, others, or the world.
   - **Hyperarousal:** Experiencing heightened anxiety, irritability, hypervigilance, exaggerated startle response, and difficulty sleeping or concentrating.
   - **Emotional Reactivity:** Experiencing strong and intense emotional reactions, including anger, fear, guilt, or shame, often triggered by reminders of the trauma.
2. **Impact on Functioning:** PTSD can significantly affect various aspects of life, including relationships, work or school performance, social interactions, and overall quality of life. It can lead to difficulties in maintaining healthy relationships, holding employment, or engaging in daily activities.
3. **Co-Occurring Conditions:** PTSD frequently co-occurs with other mental health conditions such as depression, anxiety disorders, substance use disorders, and sleep disturbances.
4. **Onset and Duration:** While some individuals may develop symptoms shortly after the traumatic event, for others, symptoms may not emerge until months or even years later. The duration of PTSD varies; some individuals experience symptoms for a few months, while others may have a chronic course of symptoms lasting years.

In order to be diagnosed with PTSD your symptoms would have to go on for several weeks and have a significant impact on your life. These symptoms may develop while you are undergoing treatment or they may develop in the weeks and months after treatment has finished. It is not uncommon for clients to present to the doctor with symptoms of emotional and physical distress after their treatment diagnosis and also after their treatment has finished. They may report ongoing psychological distress that results in panic and anxiety or depression and they may feel guilty for these feelings given that treatment has gone well. In many cases people have simply had no time to manage the emotions associated with their diagnosis they had to “box” them up and “get on with treatment”. However, emotional distress has a nasty way of turning up when we least expect it, if it does show up it is time to get help. If you are noticing that you have symptoms consistent with what has been discussed here then please go to your GP and see what services you can access and help you can get. There is no point leaving it. In my experience as a therapist the longer you leave it the worse it gets and I promise you it is very unlikely that your distress will “go away” by itself.

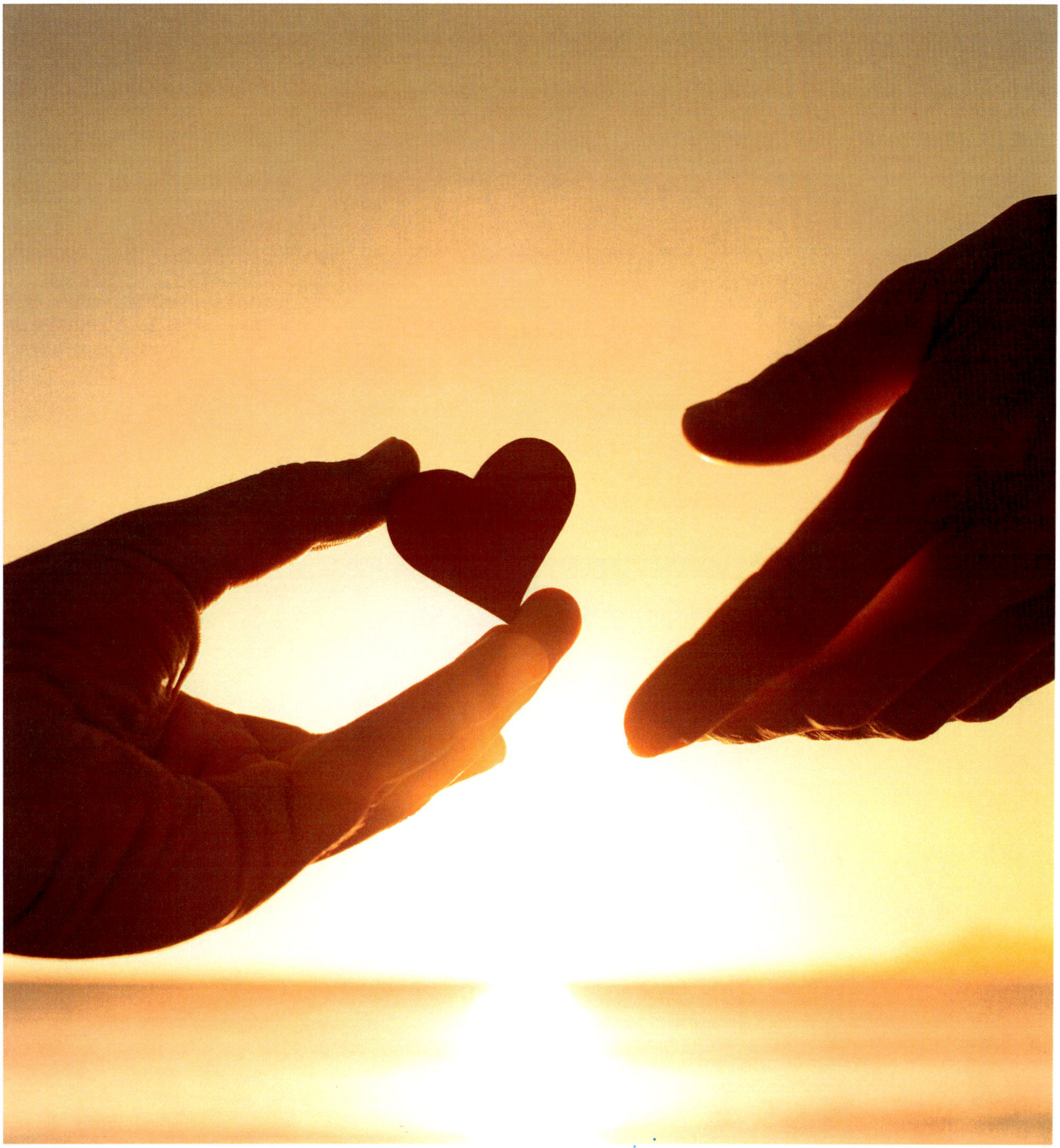

# COMPLEX-PTSD

Complex post-traumatic stress disorder (C-PTSD) is a psychological condition that can develop in individuals who have experienced prolonged and repeated trauma, typically within the context of interpersonal relationships, such as childhood abuse, neglect, or ongoing domestic violence. This is also complicated when there is a diagnosis such as cancer in addition to these traumas. It is not always the case that someone with cancer will develop complex trauma but it is definitely something to be aware of and you could develop it as a result of the treatment itself. C-PTSD is not yet officially recognized as a distinct diagnosis in the Diagnostic and Statistical Manual of Mental Disorders (DSM-5), but it is often used to describe a set of symptoms that extend beyond the criteria for PTSD. Here are some key features and symptoms associated with C-PTSD:

1. **Prolonged Trauma:** C-PTSD is typically associated with chronic and long-lasting traumatic experiences, often occurring during childhood or in situations involving abuse and ongoing life threatening situations such as repeated treatments.
2. **Emotional Dysregulation:** Individuals with C-PTSD often experience difficulties regulating their emotions. This may manifest as intense and overwhelming emotional reactions, mood swings, emotional numbness, and difficulty identifying and expressing emotions.
3. **Distorted Self-Perception:** C-PTSD can lead to a negative and distorted view of oneself. Individuals may experience feelings of shame, guilt, and a pervasive sense of worthlessness. They may also struggle with a fragmented or inconsistent sense of self.
4. **Difficulty Forming Relationships:** C-PTSD can impair the individual's ability to form and maintain healthy relationships. Trust issues, fear of abandonment, difficulties with intimacy and emotional connection, and a tendency to repeat patterns of abuse in your relationships.
5. **Changes in Beliefs and Perception:** C-PTSD can lead to significant changes in how individuals perceive themselves, others, and the world. They may develop negative beliefs about trust, safety, and the intentions of others. They may also experience feelings of helplessness, hopelessness, and a loss of meaning or purpose in life.
6. **Hypervigilance and Sensory Sensitivity:** Individuals with C-PTSD may be in a constant state of hyperarousal and hypervigilance, always anticipating danger. They may be easily startled, have exaggerated startle responses, and be highly sensitive to sensory stimuli.
7. **Dissociation:** Dissociative symptoms, such as feeling disconnected from one's body or emotions, memory gaps, or experiencing episodes of "spacing out," (dissociation) can be present in C-PTSD. This is a powerful coping mechanism.

In order to be diagnosed with CPTSD, you would need to be experiencing all of the symptoms of PTSD as well as additional symptoms which impact quality of life.

# SYMPTOMS OF CPTSD

While C-PTSD is not typically associated with a specific traumatic event like PTSD, it can result from ongoing trauma, such as childhood abuse, domestic violence, or prolonged exposure to stressful situations such as prolonged or difficult cancer treatments.

When considering cancer in the context of C-PTSD, several factors may contribute to the development or exacerbation of C-PTSD symptoms:

1. **Trauma of Diagnosis and Treatment:** The diagnosis of cancer and subsequent treatment can be traumatic experiences, particularly for individuals who have a history of trauma. The physical and emotional challenges associated with cancer treatment can trigger memories of past trauma and exacerbate C-PTSD symptoms.
2. **Loss of Control:** Cancer diagnosis and treatment often involve a loss of control over one's body and circumstances. For individuals with a history of trauma, feelings of powerlessness and helplessness can be particularly triggering and may worsen C-PTSD symptoms.
3. **Medical Trauma:** Some cancer patients experience medical trauma as a result of invasive procedures, complications, or negative interactions with healthcare providers. Medical trauma can compound existing trauma and contribute to the development of C-PTSD symptoms.
4. **Fear of Recurrence and Uncertainty:** Even after successful treatment, cancer survivors may experience ongoing fear of recurrence and uncertainty about the future. For individuals with C-PTSD, this fear and uncertainty can be especially distressing and may trigger symptoms such as hypervigilance, anxiety, and intrusive memories.
5. **Impact on Relationships:** Cancer can strain relationships with partners, family members, and friends. For individuals with a history of trauma, relational difficulties can be particularly triggering and may exacerbate symptoms of C-PTSD, such as difficulties with trust, intimacy, and communication.

These symptoms may be present and certainly be more prevalent in some rather than others. Addressing C-PTSD in the context of cancer requires a comprehensive approach that considers both the physical and emotional aspects of the illness. This may involve trauma-informed therapy, support groups, mindfulness practices, medication, and other interventions aimed at promoting healing and resilience. It's essential for individuals with cancer and C-PTSD to receive compassionate and integrated care that acknowledges the complex interplay between physical health, mental health, and trauma history.

**NOTES:**
DO YOU RECOGNISE ANY OF THESE SYMPTOMS IN YOURSELF? IF YOU DO WRITE DOWN THE ONES THAT YOU THINK YOU HAVE.

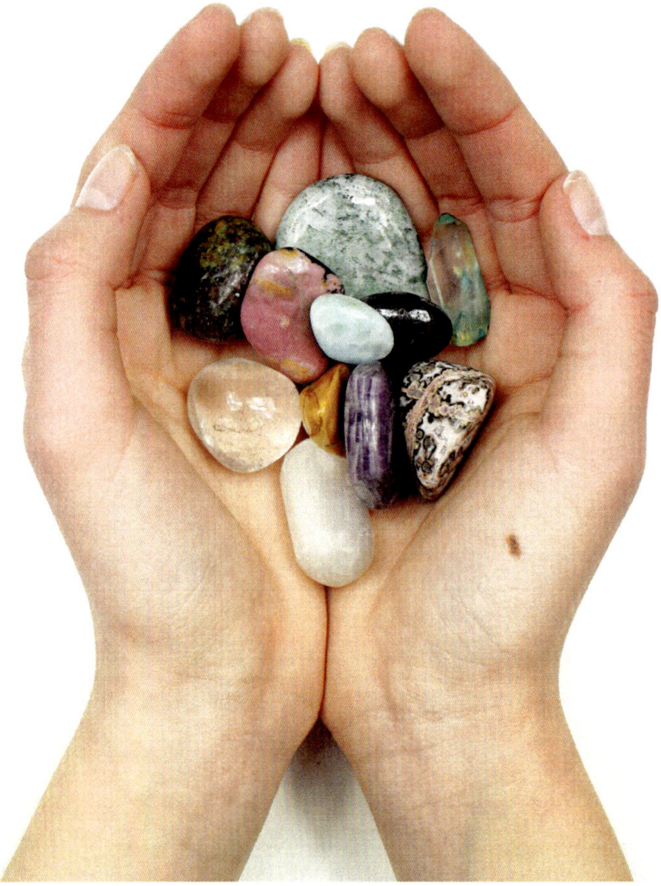

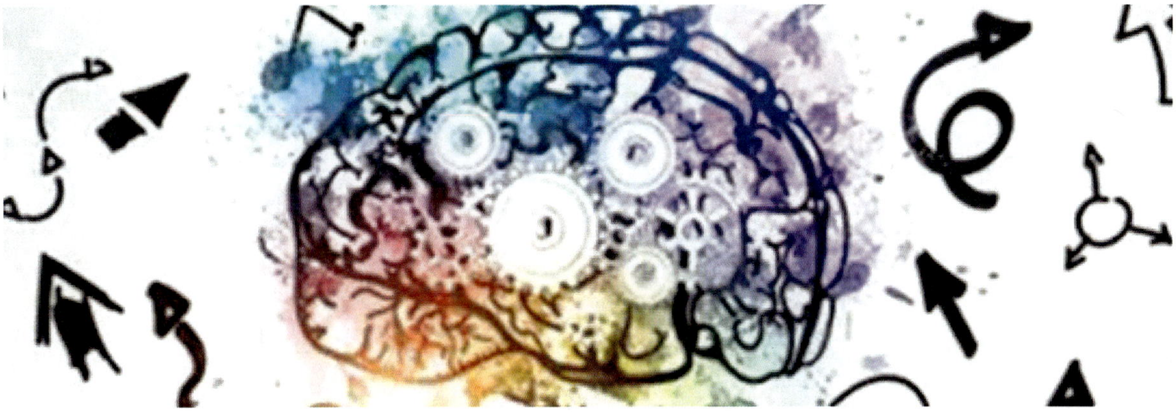

# PSYCHOEDUCATION

It is important before you go any further that you understand exactly what is happening with your body when you experience PTSD or CPTSD symptoms. If you don't understand the physical elements of what is happening to you it makes it harder to understand how to use strategies in the right ways at the right times to calm yourself down and also how to manage your thoughts and feelings.

Often when we experience trauma our bodies respond to even the slightest triggers with a very extreme physical response which can feel terrifying and we feel out of control. We aren't out of control but we need to learn what is going on so we feel less frightened and we can learn ways to manage our extreme emotional reactions.

When something out of the ordinary occurs and you are traumatised by an overwhelming event (e.g. a diagnosis) or by being repeatedly subjected to distress (e.g. medical treatments), your natural coping mechanism can become overloaded. This overloading can result in experiences remaining frozen in your brain or being "unprocessed". Such unprocessed memories and feelings are stored in the limbic system of your brain in a "raw" and emotional form, rather than in a verbal "story" mode. This limbic system maintains traumatic memories in an isolated memory (or imprint) network that is associated with emotions and physical sensations, and these memories are disconnected from the brain's cortex where we use language to store memories. The limbic system's traumatic memories can be continually triggered when you experience events similar to the difficult experiences you have been

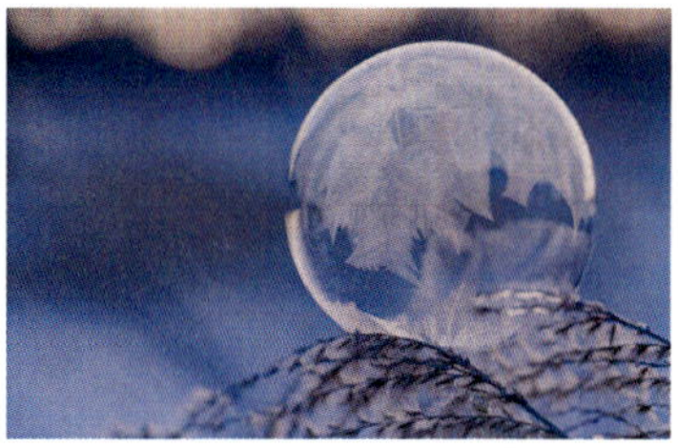

through. Often the memory itself is long forgotten, but the painful feelings such as anxiety, panic, anger or despair are continually triggered in the present. Your ability to live in the present and learn from new experiences can therefore become negatively impacted.

What happens to me when I get Anxious?

When triggered by something unexpected the brain automatically engages an emergency "hot line" to the fear centre in the brain (the red arrow points to the spot!)

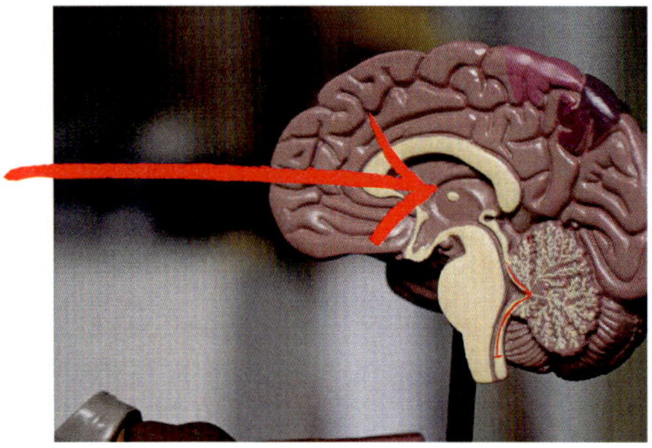

Only after the fear response is activated does the conscious mind start to work. Some sensory information, rather than travelling directly to the Amygdala (which is a processing centre for our emotions), this information takes a different route stopping first at the processing hub for sensory information and then the cortex (the outer layer of the brain cells which is responsible for problem solving). The cortex analyses the raw data streaming in through the senses and decides if the information requires a fear response. If the brain "decides" a fear response is needed to protect us from danger, the cortex signals the Amygdala and the body stays on alert. In other words the brain tells itself to stay on high alert to danger.

When triggered the brain sends messages to the body to flight to get rid of the perceived danger or to fight which then results in physical symptoms (heart rate increases, stress hormones, digestion shutdown, hypervigilance and distress).

In this state people act on instinct to get away from what they think is a threat. In this way the brain and body "acts first" and "thinks later" about the consequences.

When we are born our system is not fully developed and so this system is there to help us get our needs met. As an adult, we have learned to assess the information being sent to the frontal lobe (problem solving area of the brain) and assess the situation to make a decision about how to act based on previous experience. We also know the ways that help to settle ourselves down and feel less anxious. By age 10 we can make decisions quickly about our safety. This is based on our experience and "learning" what is a threat and what is not.

Traumatic stress can be seen as part of a normal human response to intense experiences. While most people recover in the first few months from something that is upsetting, for some the symptoms do not seem to resolve quickly and, may continue to cause problems for the rest of the person's life. It is also common for symptoms to vary in intensity over time. Some people go for long periods without any significant problems, only to relapse when they have to deal with other major life stress or they are reminded of the trauma. In rare cases, the symptoms may not appear for months, or even years, after the trauma.

After a trauma such as PTSD (single event) the brain has to contend with a lot of new information that is hard to accept or understand.

When people experience
a trauma, the event keeps coming back into their mind in an attempt to make sense of what happened or try to rationalise the irrational. This is the body's natural way of trying to "deal with", or come to terms with, difficult experiences and seems to work well for many stressful life events. However, due to the high level of distress associated with memories of more severe trauma, the thoughts and feelings might be pushed away as a way to "protect" the person from something frightening and upsetting. It is "protective" in the short term and "maladaptive" in the long run as we learn to "avoid" things and is especially problematic if we "avoid" treatment for our cancer.

The result is that, whilst the memory may be supressed for a while, the distressing memory keeps coming back. This results in a cycle of being triggered by memories and then pushing frightening memories away until we are triggered again. This cycle is exhausting and feels a bit like a volcano building up.......until it "blows" and then the cycle starts all over again.

Throughout this alternating between short bursts of painful memories and periods of avoidance and numbing, is the sense of feeling "on edge" all the time. The traumatised person has been through an event that threatened their life, or the life of someone else, so the mind and body are on "high alert" to protect the person from dangers in the future.

The brain and body are engaged in "overdrive to protect the individual from danger" In addition, the threat detection system becomes so efficient that it is constantly "going off" signalling danger and alerts when there is no danger. As a result this constant state of alarm interferes with the person's capacity to live a normal and happy life.

Traumatic stress reactions, are important and they serve a protective function to "keep us safe from harm" and most of the time the reactions we develop as survival mechanisms are helpful and valuable until they become overwhelming. As a result, treatment for trauma centres around understanding and knowing where our symptoms come from and why. Once we recognise where these symptoms come from, it is easier to understand our stress reactions. The hard part is learning to let go of our "protective" reactions now that they are interfering with quality of life. After all until these reactions interfered with quality of life they were very effective at protecting us from thinking about the thing that hurt us physically or emotionally or both. This is especially true if this system protected us during treatment for cancer.

When we have CPTSD there is another layer of complication to our responses to trauma.

Polyvagal theory emphasizes the evolutionary development of two systems: the parasympathetic nervous system which is ultimately connected to the vagal nerve and the sympathetic nervous system. Each has its own function, and cause the body to react differently before, during, and after a traumatic or stressful event. If these two systems become damaged from excessive and recurrent trauma, a break down occurs and mental illnesses such as CPTSD and anxiety disorders may result.

The sympathetic nervous system gets the body ready for the fight/flight/freeze response. With the fight or flight response, the sympathetic nervous system begins revving up the heartbeat and blood pressure and stealing blood from the body to make muscles ready to run.
If there is nowhere to run and no hope of escape, the sympathetic nervous system will cause the person to freeze or collapse (both forms of dissociation). The parasympathetic nervous system is a calming force, that when kicked in, allows the heart rate and blood pressure to lower, calming down the body after a traumatic event. If the sympathetic nervous system is hyper-aroused then the body suffers from a lack of adequate blood supply as the person is always ready to flee or fight. This damages the person's ability to calm down after being triggered by something that even barely resembles the danger that caused the psychological injury.

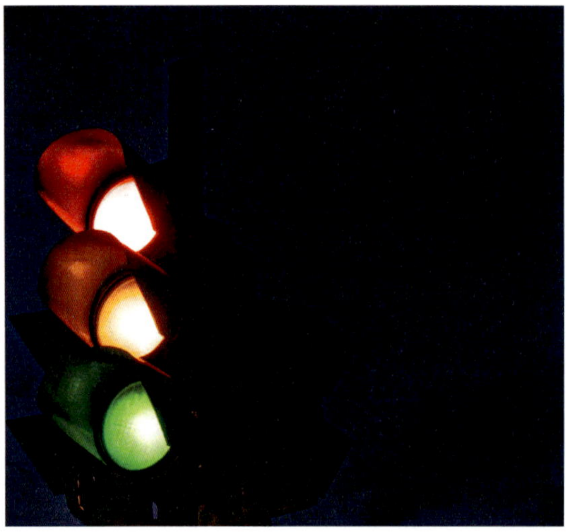

The leading cause of damage to the nervous system is the overwhelming and chronic washing of the brain by stress hormones brought on by severe and repeated trauma. This is most often associated with childhood abuse but make no mistake, repeated trauma of any kind that impacts your sense of powerlessness can cause you to experience trauma.

Stress hormones are notoriously known to damage a child's brain including the vagal nerve and both the parasympathetic and sympathetic nervous systems.

So basically this means that you need to learn different ways to manage your nervous system and how to stay mindful of your symptoms and use skills to help you stay in a "regulated" zone.

Think of your nervous system as a traffic light. The green zone is the Ventral Vagal zone and this is when we are able to be socially connected and feel safe. The next zone is when the sympathetic nervous system has been activated and we are in Flight (move away) or Fight (movement towards). When in Fight or Flight our system is designed to get away from the bad thing that could hurt us or fight the threat. Normally we would expend energy and our nervous system would settle back down to the green zone. EXCEPT when we have experienced a trauma and we are unable to regulate ourselves again. The third zone is the red zone and this is Dorsal Vagal. This state is an EMERGENCY state and the body freezes and we experience immobility. In this state we can become dissociated, numb, helpless, shut down and feel trapped in our extreme physical distress.

Most people only experience the Dorsal or Freeze state in an extreme situation. However, if you have complex trauma or CPTSD you may experience this state very easily and you can be easily triggered to get to this heightened state of arousal and it is very difficult to "come back down". Some people even state that they cycle between the Sympathetic state and the Dorsal state and they almost never know what the Ventral Vagal state feels like. In other words they don't know what "relaxed" feels like in the body.

The good news is that with the right treatment you can learn to manage your system and not let your physical symptoms take over........ this is especially important if you need to cope with treatment.

Treatment for trauma typically involves an individualized approach that addresses the trauma history, symptoms, and functional impairments. It may include various therapies like trauma-focused therapy (e.g. prolonged exposure therapy, cognitive processing therapy), dialectical behaviour therapy (DBT), eye movement desensitization and reprocessing (EMDR), as well as additional therapies to address emotional dysregulation, self-esteem, and relationship difficulties. Treatment is not a one size "fits all".

Medication may also be considered to manage specific symptoms like depression, anxiety, or sleep disturbances. Treatment for PTSD typically involves a combination of therapy, medication, and self-help strategies. Further your doctor may need be aware of your distress to properly direct you to the right treatment to manage your symptoms. These may include:

**Psychotherapy:** Various forms of psychotherapy, such as cognitive-behavioural therapy (CBT), are effective in treating PTSD. CBT helps individuals identify and change negative thought patterns and behaviours associated with the traumatic event. Exposure therapy, a type of CBT, involves gradually exposing the person to memories, situations, or objects associated with the trauma in a safe and controlled environment, helping to reduce fear and anxiety.

**Eye Movement Desensitization and Reprocessing (EMDR):** EMDR is a specialized form of therapy that helps individuals process traumatic memories and reduce their emotional impact. It involves focusing on the traumatic event while engaging in bilateral stimulation, such as eye movements or hand taps, to help the brain reprocess the memories in a healthier way.

**Group Therapy:** Participating in group therapy can provide a supportive environment where individuals with PTSD can share their experiences, learn from others, and gain coping strategies.

Supportive Relationships: Having a strong support system of family, friends, or support groups can be beneficial for individuals with PTSD. Loved ones can provide understanding, empathy, and practical support, which can aid in the recovery process.

Lifestyle Changes: Engaging in self-care activities, such as regular exercise, practicing relaxation techniques (e.g., deep breathing, meditation), getting enough sleep, and avoiding alcohol and drugs, can help manage PTSD symptoms. Additionally, avoiding triggers and creating a safe and structured environment can contribute to overall well-being.

Medications: Antidepressant medications, such as selective serotonin reuptake inhibitors (SSRIs) or serotonin-norepinephrine reuptake inhibitors (SNRIs), are often prescribed to help manage the symptoms of PTSD. These medications can help alleviate depression, anxiety, and improve sleep patterns.

**It's important to note that treatment for PTSD or CPTSD should be individualized, and what works for one person may not work for another. The other important piece of information is that an approach that combines evidence based treatments can work together to provide a way forward. While some people only need to deal with aspects of their trauma once, others may need to accept that it can take time to work through many levels of trauma to find a way forward. Everyone is different...........BUT everyone is worth the effort**

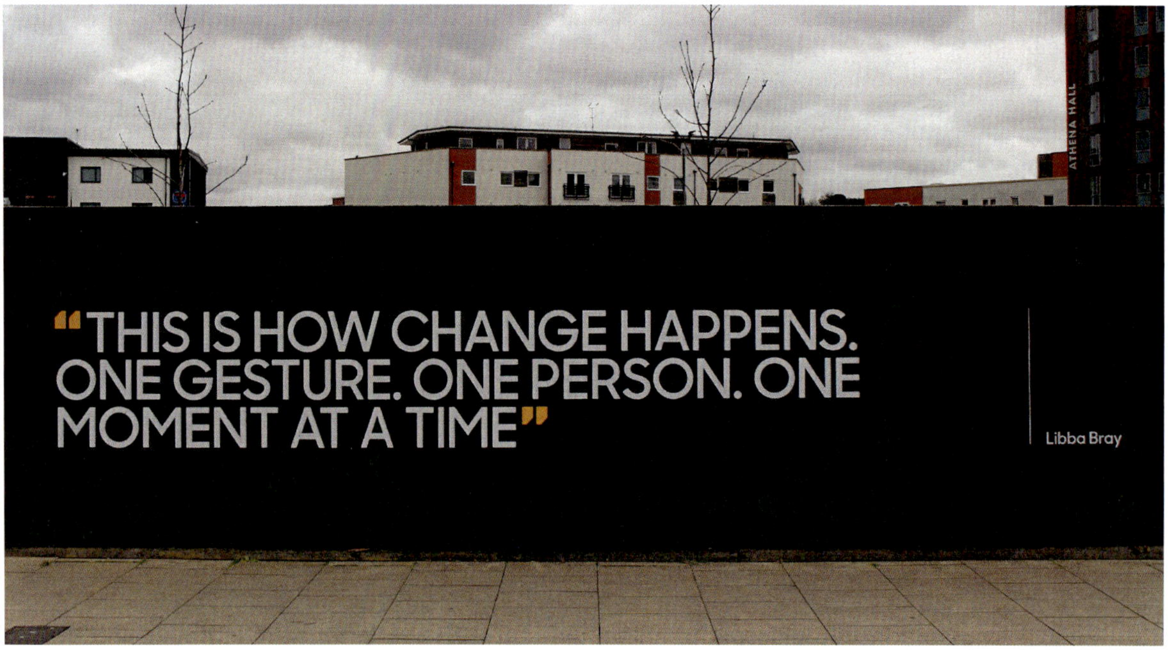

# STRATEGIES

A strategy is a plan to achieve one or more long term goals to be used in times of uncertainty. If undergoing treatment for cancer is not a time to use strategies to cope then I don't know when is! In the next section there are a group of strategies designed to help you. These strategies are designed to help you to think about how you would like to try and take back some control and what you may need in the coming months or even after your treatment has finished. There are also strategies to help you cope when you feel overwhelmed and experience difficult moments as you are undergoing your treatment. There is also space for you to add things that work for you in the moment or strategies that you may have discussed with your therapist. These strategies with time will help you to know what to do when you feel out of control and rather than do something that will make things worse, you can have a choice to do things that help you to live your best life even though you are going through one of the most difficult times in your life........

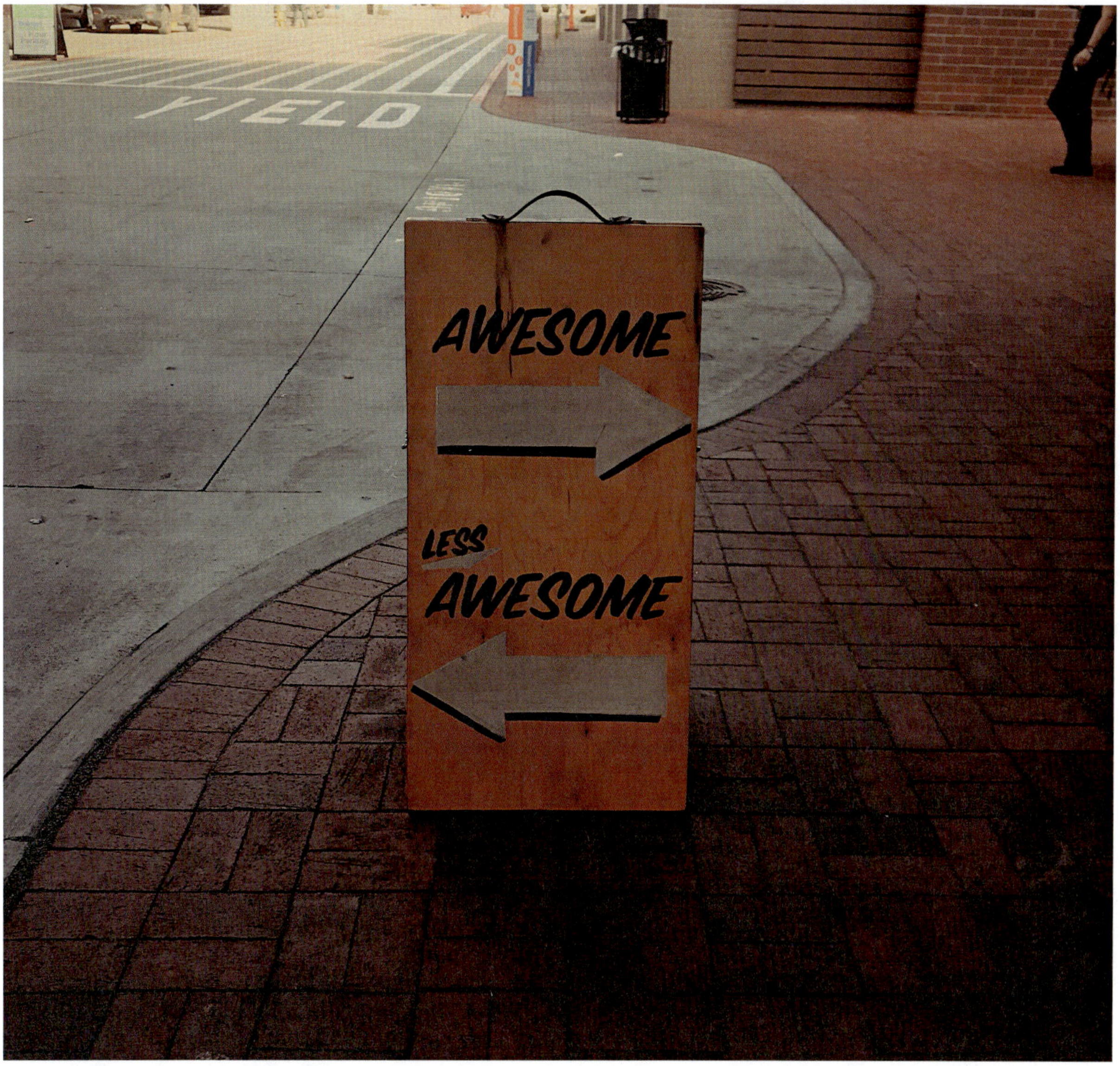

# WHY ARE STRATEGIES HELPFUL?

Well bluntly you are about to go through a tough time and you are going to have to focus on what is important which is treatment. Your body needs all of its reserves to help get you well and when we are scared we spiral and our anxiety can take over....which is not going to be helpful. By learning what is going on in your body and working out ways to deal with all of the anxious feelings it will help you to cope when things feel out of control. You have quite a way to go and your head needs to help your body stay calm. Over the next few pages we are going to be looking at some things you can do in the moment when the anxiety threatens to take over and make us feel totally out of our depth.

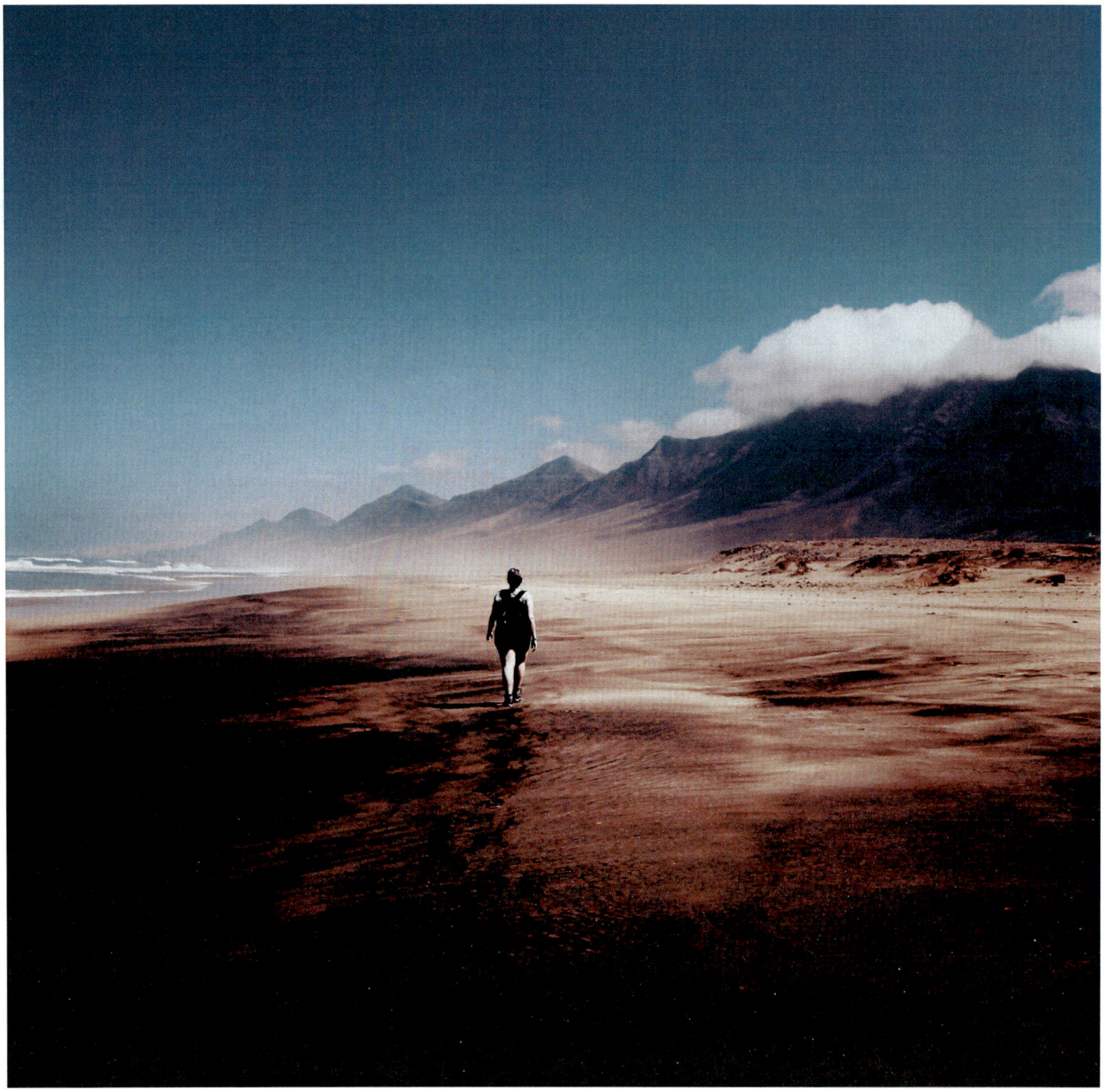

# VISUALISATION

Visualization is a cognitive technique that involves creating mental images or scenarios to achieve a desired outcome. It's a powerful tool that can be used for various purposes, including relaxation, goal-setting, performance improvement, and managing stress. This is really important right now as you can start to build your own confidence and how you would like things to be. I have broken this up into two parts, the first is that you have the different ways it can be used but the second is how it can be used specifically with your treatment. Here are some ways visualization can be applied:

- **Relaxation and Stress Reduction:**
  - Find a quiet and comfortable space. Close your eyes and visualize a peaceful scene, such as a tranquil beach or a calming forest. Imagine the sights, sounds, and smells of this serene environment. Focusing on positive imagery can help reduce stress and promote relaxation.
- **Goal Setting and Achievement:**
  - Envision your goals as already accomplished. Picture the steps you took to achieve them and the positive outcomes. Visualizing success can enhance motivation and build confidence.
- **Performance Enhancement:**
  - Mentally rehearse and imagine yourself successfully completing a task, or treatment.
- **Overcoming Challenges:**
  - When facing challenges or obstacles, visualize yourself overcoming them. Picture the steps you need to take and imagine the positive emotions associated with overcoming adversity. This can help shift your mindset toward problem-solving.
- **Positive Affirmations:**
  - Combine visualization with positive affirmations. Picture yourself achieving your goals while repeating positive statements about your abilities and worth. This can reinforce a positive self-image.
- **Pain Management:**
  - Visualization can be used as part of pain management techniques. Focus on imagining a place or activity that brings you comfort and joy while breathing out deeply and letting go of tension.
- **Creativity Boost:**
  - Visualize creative ideas or solutions to problems. Picture the details and intricacies of your innovative thoughts. This can enhance creativity and inspire new perspectives.
  - You might want to write these down or start a journal. Putting your ideas down might help you when you are feeling unwell from treatment.

NOTES

- **Behavioural Change:**
  - Use visualization to imagine yourself making positive changes in your habits or lifestyle. Visualize each of the steps involved and the benefits that will come from these changes.
- **Future Planning:**
  - Picture your ideal future. Envision the life you want to lead, the relationships you want to cultivate, and the accomplishments you aim to achieve. This can provide a clear vision and motivation for working towards your aspirations.

**Remember that effective visualization involves engaging multiple senses and emotions. The more vivid and detailed your mental images, the more powerful the impact of visualization can be. Additionally, consistent practice writing them down and reviewing them regularly is often key to reaping the full benefits of this technique.**

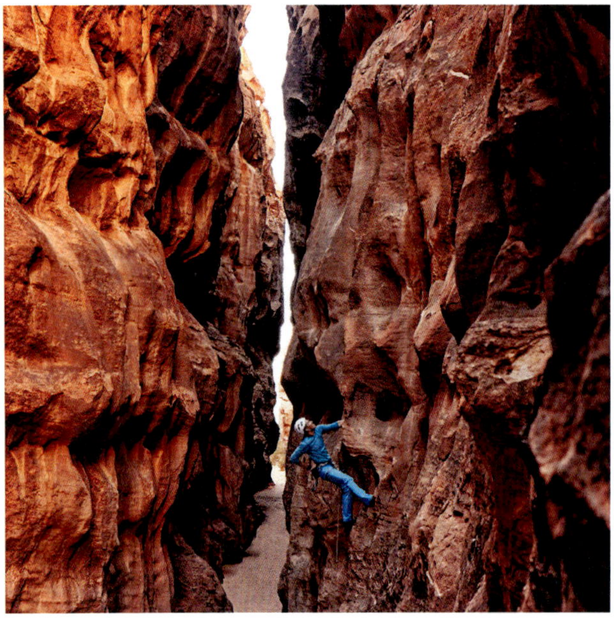

# TREATMENT VISUALISATION

Visualization, or guided imagery, is a relaxation technique that involves creating mental images to promote relaxation, reduce stress, and enhance well-being. While visualization is not a substitute for medical treatment, it can complement traditional cancer therapies by supporting overall emotional and psychological health. Here are some visualization techniques that may be helpful for you:

- **Healing Imagery:** Visualize your body's innate healing abilities. Close your eyes and imagine a healing light or energy flowing through your body, targeting areas affected by cancer cells and promoting healing and restoration.
- **Immune Support:** Picture your immune system as a powerful army, actively identifying and eliminating cancer cells. Visualize your immune cells as strong, vigilant defenders, working tirelessly to protect your body from illness.
- **Comfort and Relaxation:** Imagine yourself in a peaceful and serene environment, such as a tranquil beach, forest, or garden. Focus on the sights, sounds, and sensations of this imaginary place, allowing yourself to feel calm, relaxed, and at ease.
- **Pain Management:** Visualize pain as a sensation that can be controlled and minimized. Picture yourself breathing in healing energy and exhaling tension and discomfort. Imagine it melting like ice under the warm sun.
- **Treatment Efficacy:** Visualize your cancer treatment (such as chemotherapy, radiation, or surgery) as a powerful force targeting and destroying cancer cells. Picture the treatment reaching the intended target with precision and effectiveness, shrinking tumours and restoring health.
- **Emotional Support:** Visualize yourself surrounded by a supportive network of loved ones, friends, and healthcare providers. Imagine their presence, love, and encouragement as sources of strength and comfort .
- **Future Wellness:** Envision yourself in the future, healthy, and thriving. Picture yourself engaging in activities you enjoy, pursuing your passions, and living a fulfilling life beyond cancer treatment. This might be the most important "visualisation" of all.

When practicing visualization, find a quiet and comfortable space where you won't be interrupted. Close your eyes, take slow, deep breaths, and allow yourself to immerse fully in the visualizations. It's essential to approach visualization with an open mind and a willingness to explore the healing power of your imagination. If you find it challenging to visualize images, you can also focus on sensations, emotions, or affirmations related to healing and well-being. Additionally, consider working with a qualified healthcare professional or therapist experienced in visualization techniques.

# VISUALISATION......

### What kind of life do you want ?

Think about the kind of life you want. It is very important that you know why you are doing the treatment and what is important to you.

This is the first step in preparing your self for what is to come.  A useful thing to try is to visualise your life as you want it to be and what your life will look like after cancer.  What are you working towards? What is important to you? Who is important to you?  How do you want to live It is common for a diagnosis of cancer to really make us stop and think about who we are and what is important to us.

In the notes space on the next page write down a clear picture of what you want your life to look like. If it is too hard to write a clear picture just put down some ideas and come back to the clear picture when you can.

If you are able form the clear picture in your mind, then imagine as much as you can. Imagine where you would like to be living and why? Think about the kinds of friends you want and what kind of job you might like? Think about what are the things that make you happy and what you enjoy doing?

When you form the clear picture in your head sit with it for a moment and let the clear picture form all the colours. Picture the place you are in as clearly as you can. See yourself in the picture and note how you look and what you are wearing. Note to yourself who is in the picture with you is it a dog? or friend? or family member?

Once the picture is really clear start to write it down on the next page. This will be important for the future. When you feel low or you are struggling you can come back to the note you write and remind yourself why you are doing the treatment and why.

Visualization is a technique that involves creating mental images or scenarios to achieve a desired outcome and in this case it is getting through the treatment. It's a powerful tool that can be used for various purposes, including relaxation, goal-setting, and managing stress. This skill is also a wonderful motivational tool.  It reminds us when we are in a low place and having a moment during our cancer journey and what we will do differently in the future.

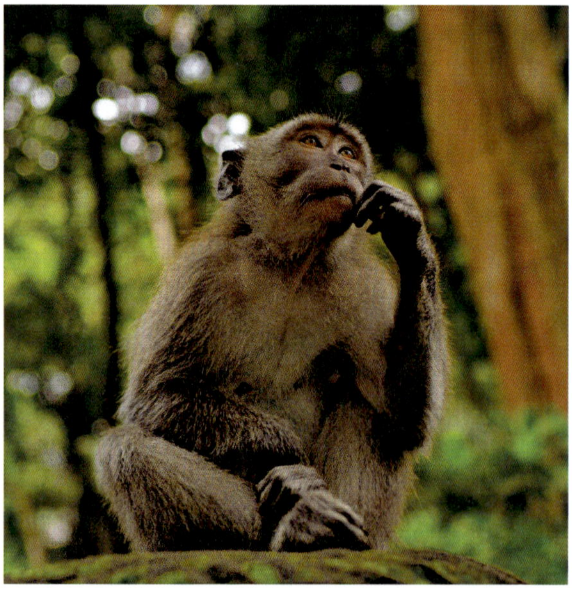

# MY IDEAL LIFE

# TYPES OF STRATEGIES

A strategy is a plan or course of action designed to achieve a specific goal or objective. It is a systematic approach that outlines the steps and resources required to accomplish a desired outcome. Strategies are tools that can be used to help you manage your emotional distress especially during treatment and when you are feeling panicked or anxious. There are a number of different strategies to help with your distress and some of these we have already discussed earlier:

1. **Education and self-awareness:** Learn about your treatments and how they might affect you. Understanding the procedures symptoms, triggers, and common reactions can help you gain insight into your own experiences and develop effective coping strategies.
2. **Establish a support system:** Build a support network of friends, family, and fellow survivors who can provide understanding, empathy, and encouragement.
3. **Practice self-care:** Engage in activities that promote physical and emotional well-being. This may include regular exercise, healthy eating, sufficient sleep, relaxation techniques (such as deep breathing, meditation, or mindfulness), and engaging in hobbies or activities you enjoy.
4. **Develop coping strategies:** Look at various coping mechanisms that can help you manage distressing symptoms. These may include grounding techniques, journaling, art therapy, music therapy, or engaging in activities that promote relaxation and stress reduction.
5. **Create a routine:** Establishing a structured daily routine can provide a sense of stability and control. Make sure to include activities that promote relaxation, self-care, and engagement in positive experiences.
6. **Manage triggers:** Identify specific triggers that worsen your symptoms and work on developing strategies to manage them. This may involve avoiding certain situations and by gradually exposing yourself to triggers in a controlled manner, or implementing relaxation techniques when confronted with triggers you will learn how to cope.
7. **Practice stress reduction techniques:** Regularly engage in stress reduction activities such as deep breathing exercises, progressive muscle relaxation, yoga, or mindfulness meditation. These techniques can help reduce anxiety and promote a sense of calm.

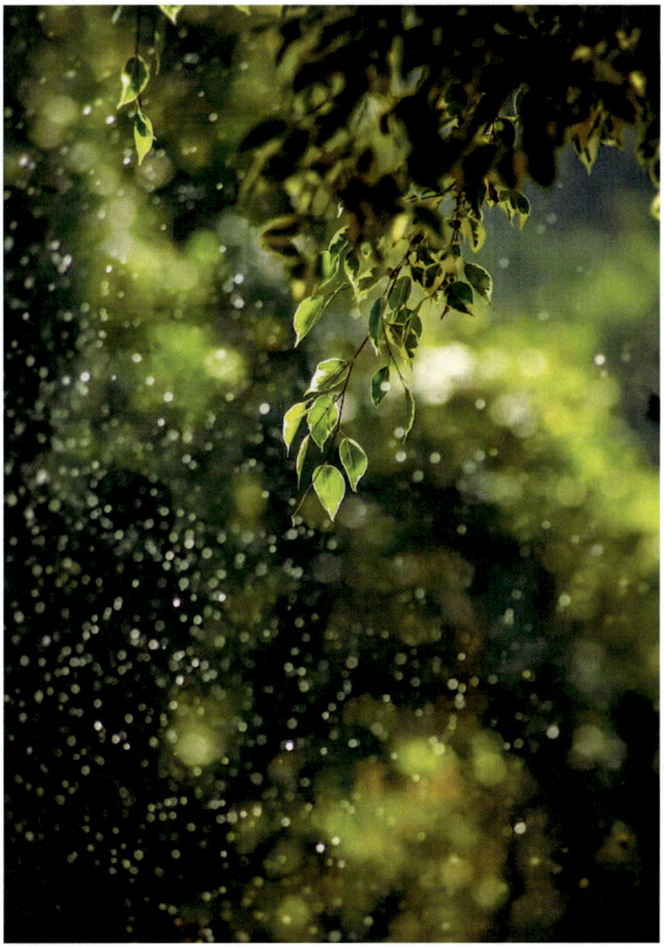

Part of the process of coping with difficult emotions is starting with knowing how your body reacts to anxiety or distress ....write your symptoms in the checklist.....if you can identify how your body reacts to stress those symptoms become your warning system to act or use a strategy...........

# SYMPTOM

# CHECKLIST

THESE ARE THE SYMPTOMS WE ARE GOING TO HELP YOU TARGET THESE ARE ALSO YOUR WARNING SIGNS WHICH TELL YOU THAT IT IS TIME TO ACT IF YOU CAN IDENTIFY THEM YOU CAN ACT ON THEM!

## BODY SYMPTOMS

- [ ] 
- [ ] 
- [ ] 
- [ ] 
- [ ] 

## THINKING

- [ ] 
- [ ] 
- [ ] 
- [ ] 
- [ ] 

## EMOTIONS

- [ ] 
- [ ] 
- [ ] 
- [ ] 
- [ ] 

## TRIGGERS

- [ ] 
- [ ] 
- [ ] 
- [ ] 
- [ ] 

# TRIGGERS

WHAT TRIGGERS ME?

| TRIGGERS | TRIGGERS |
| --- | --- |
| HOW I REACT | HOW I WANT TO REACT |

# WHY IS SELF-CARE IMPORTANT?

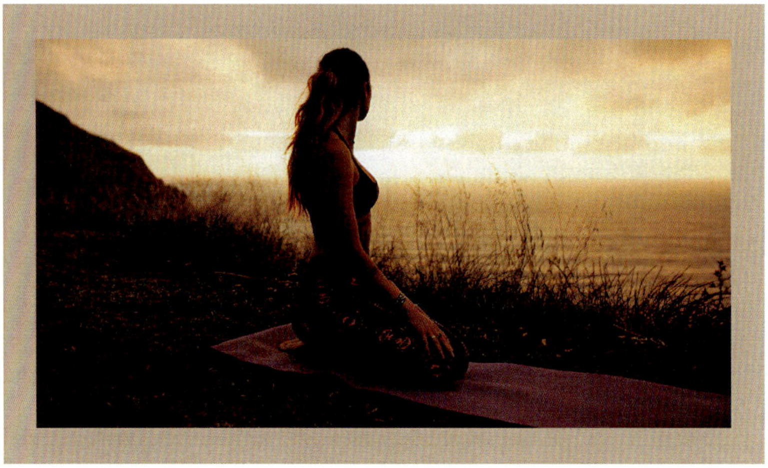

When we feel lots of different physical sensations due to triggers or when we have to do difficult things or start a new treatment regime it is easy to become overwhelmed and frightened.

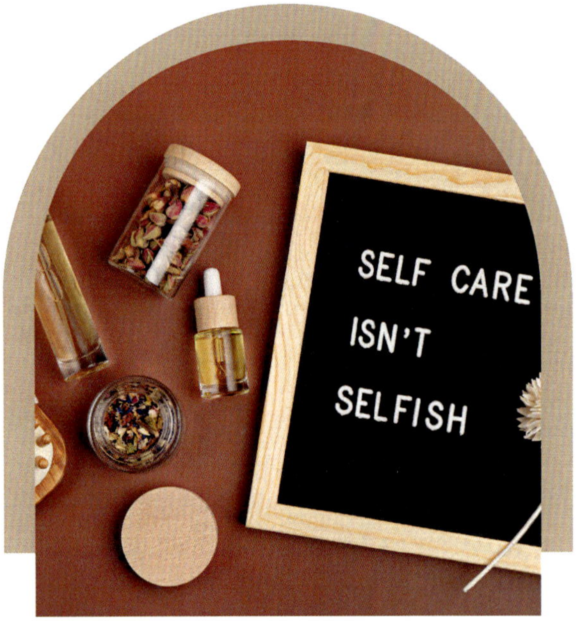


There are lots of things we can do every day to help in little ways that add to big differences in the long run. In this way we are managing the "vulnerable" factors or things that make it harder for us to cope with the emotions and physical sensations of trauma. Our vulnerable factors are things we can control. These include things such as sleep, eating well, taking medications on time, exercise and being mindful of things that make the situation worse.

# MY SELF CARE CHECKLIST

FILL IN THE CHECKLIST SPACES BELOW WITH SELF-CARE ACTIVITIES THAT YOU CAN DO IN THE MORNING AND AT NIGHT.

## MORNING SELF-CARE

- [ ] ____________________
- [ ] ____________________
- [ ] ____________________
- [ ] ____________________
- [ ] ____________________
- [ ] ____________________
- [ ] ____________________
- [ ] ____________________

## NIGHT SELF-CARE

- [ ] ____________________
- [ ] ____________________
- [ ] ____________________
- [ ] ____________________
- [ ] ____________________
- [ ] ____________________
- [ ] ____________________
- [ ] ____________________

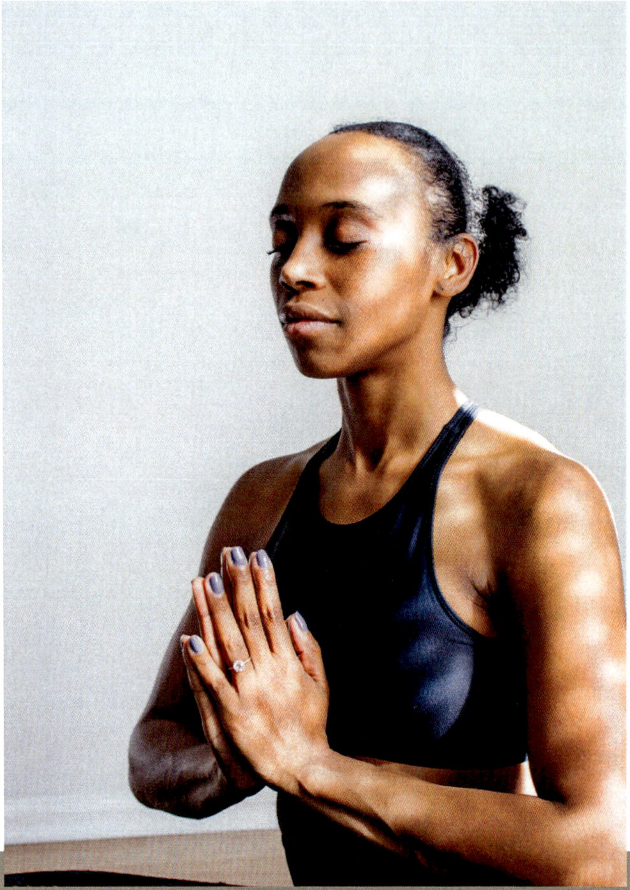

# MINDFULNESS

Mindfulness is a practice of intentionally focusing one's attention on the present moment without judgment. It involves bringing awareness to one's thoughts, emotions, bodily sensations, and the surrounding environment. Mindfulness is rooted in various contemplative traditions, particularly in Buddhism, and has gained significant attention in the fields of psychology and well-being due to its potential benefits for mental health and overall well-being.

## Choose to start right now.

*Not tomorrow, right now.*

## *Let's begin here.*

Mindfulness can be developed through formal practices like mindfulness meditation, body scan exercises, or mindful movement practices such as yoga or tai chi. Additionally, informal practices involve bringing mindfulness to daily activities such as eating, walking, or engaging in conversations. Mindfulness is a skill that can be developed over time with regular practice and patience.

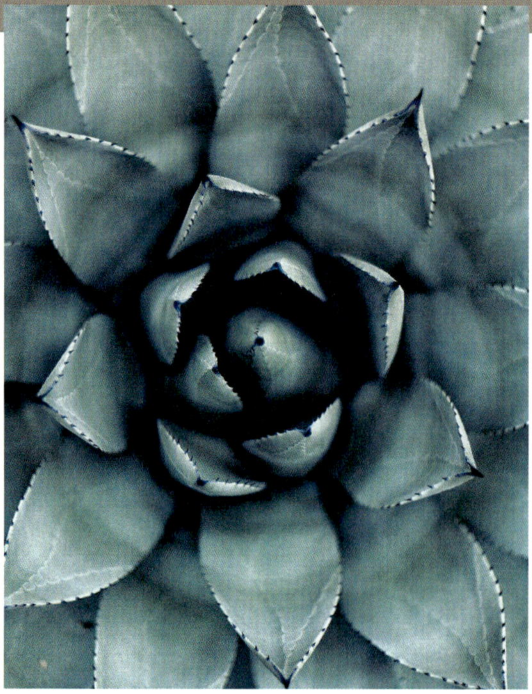

# 6 CORE MINDFULNESS SKILLS

Understanding these skills helps us to become aware of what we are already using throughout our day to help us cope with difficult things

1) **Observe:** Notice what is happening, your thoughts and feelings physical sensations, be aware and pay attention.

2) **Describe:** Write down what you have observed.

3) **Participate fully in an experience:** If you are engaged in something give it your full attention.

4) **Non-Judgemental stance:** Reduce judgements. We often label thigs as good or bad. If you feel tight in the chest you might say "I feel awful and this is embarrassing me"  a non-judgemental stance is "my chest is tight".

5) **One Mindfully:** Do one thing at a time, if you are watching TV just do that and not 3 other things at once.

6) **Effectiveness:** Do what works. If something isn't working for you, or it makes you feel worse, then try something else.

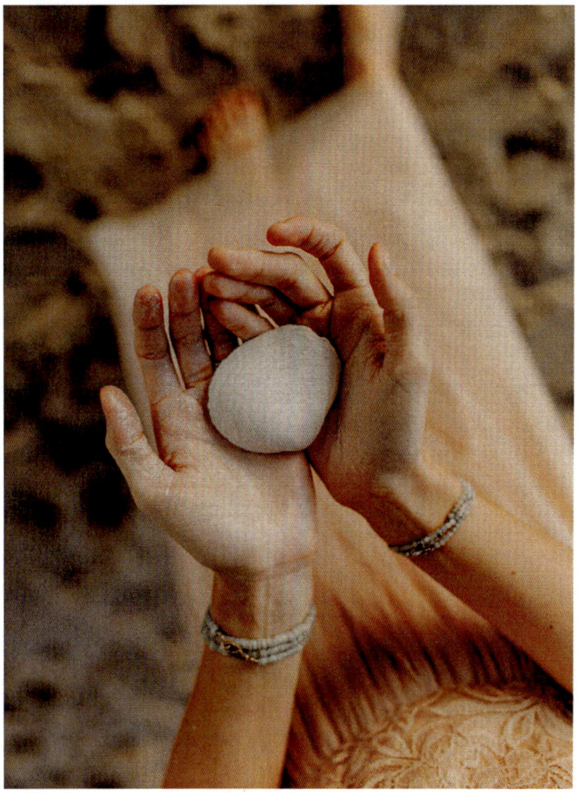

*"if something is worth doing it is with all of your heart" Buddha*

# BREATHING EXERCISE

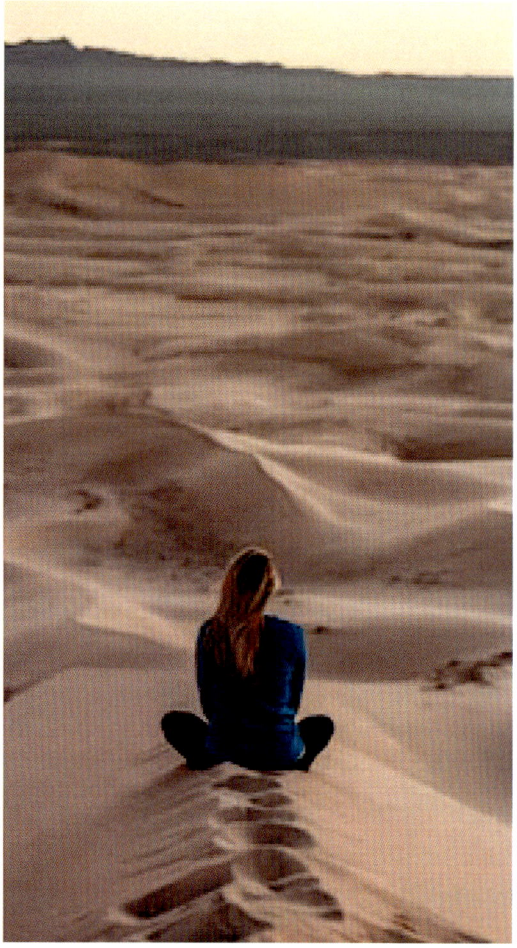

This is a great breathing exercise for when you are starting to feel the first signs of anxiety in your body.

Find quiet place where you can concentrate and feel settled.

Take a big deep breath in and hold as much air in your lungs as you can........then slowly let it out through your mouth

now breathe in..... two........ three...... hold...... and out........ two........ three...... hold......

The rate should be slow and steady with the intake matching the exhale. If you have had lots of anxiety you may find it hard at first but gradually your breaths should slow down. Aim for 10 breaths per minute.

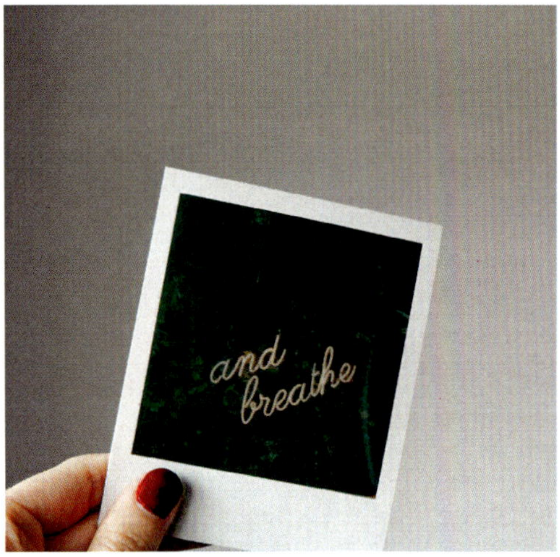


*think of something like a big rolling wave to help you with the rhythm of slow deep breaths*

# CALM PLACE

This skill is about teaching you to have a place that is safe for you. You can go there any time.

With your eyes closed, imagine yourself in a calm place....a peaceful place...this might be somewhere you visited before or somewhere you just make up in your imagination...just let the image of the place come to you...It doesn't matter what kind of place you imagine as long as it is calm, quiet, peaceful and serene...Let this be a special place for you...Somewhere you feel particularly at ease...A place where you feel safe and secure. Be at one with your surroundings...Maybe you have had a place like this in your life...Somewhere to be quiet and reflective......Somewhere special and healing for you...It could be a place from a movie or a dream...It can be somewhere you know or imagined.

Let yourself explore and experience whatever calm imaginary place you go to, as if you were there now. Notice what you see.... what you hear...the smells around you. Notice what if feels like to be there and immerse yourself in the beauty.....the peace and the security of being there.

As you explore this inner place, find a spot to be in a spot where you feel good to be in......A spot where you feel calm...centred...safe and at ease...Let yourself become comfortable in the spot...let this be your special place

Now keeping your eyes closed...can you describe this place? What do you see near you...further away....What do you hear? You can focus on particular sounds...you can add sounds if you want. What time of year is it...What time of day...What aroma do you notice...What sounds do you hear? Sensations on your skin...warm...cold...sun...shade.

As you relax and are aware of how it feels to be here....know that you can return at any time you wish...This is your calm place, your special place...A place where safety, rest and peace are always available to you at your own choosing.

What would you call this place?

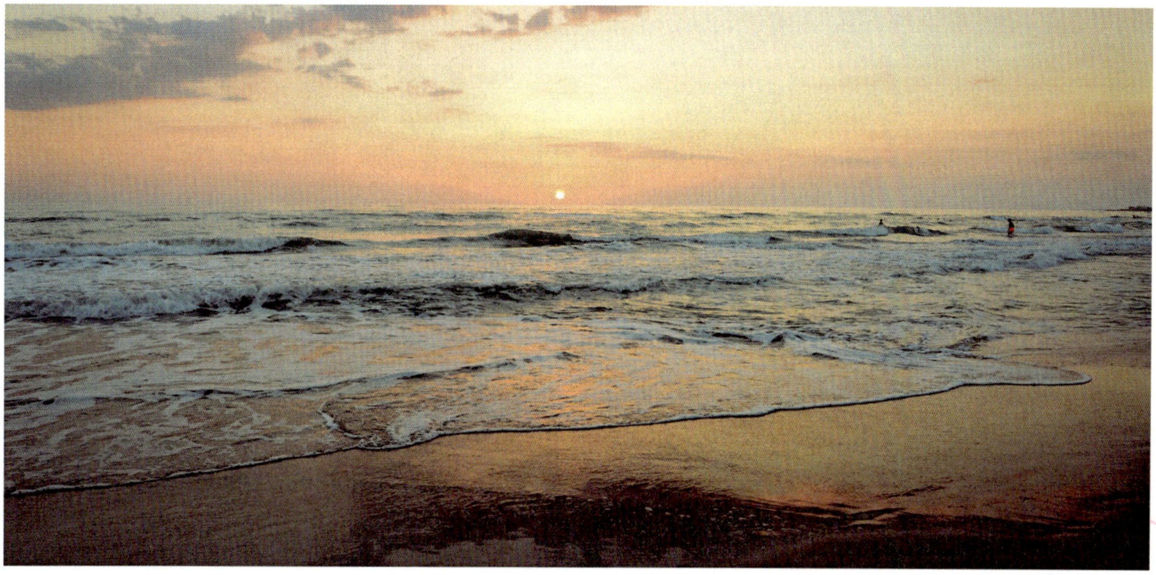

Credit Grahame Taylor Schema Therapy Training online

# HOLD!

**This is the first of three skills which help you to look at how you react when you are upset and then begin to think about how to do things differently in the future. The three skills are HOLD, FREEZE FAST and MOVE. Each of the skills can be done in any order and they are designed to be interchangeable. This first skill is HOLD. This is a way of looking at the past and how the past influences how you are responding now through either fear or past experience. In other words how the past has a hold on you!**

**History**: As yourself How is my history impacting on me now? My history is a part of me but it is also resulting in responses that are not always healthy. Remember it is in the past but still impacts you now.

**Old Reactions**: These are old patterns of behaviour and they may not help me to get my needs met in a healthy way.

**NOTES:**

How has the past got a hold on me?

Learn new Patterns: Take time to stop and reflect and to think about what you really want and if your current response is going to damage your future (e.g. getting angry at a friend to get them to do what you want or not having boundaries)

**Do**: Do something different a more healthy response. Think about the way someone you respect or admire might respond and then think about how you might be able to do that in the future.

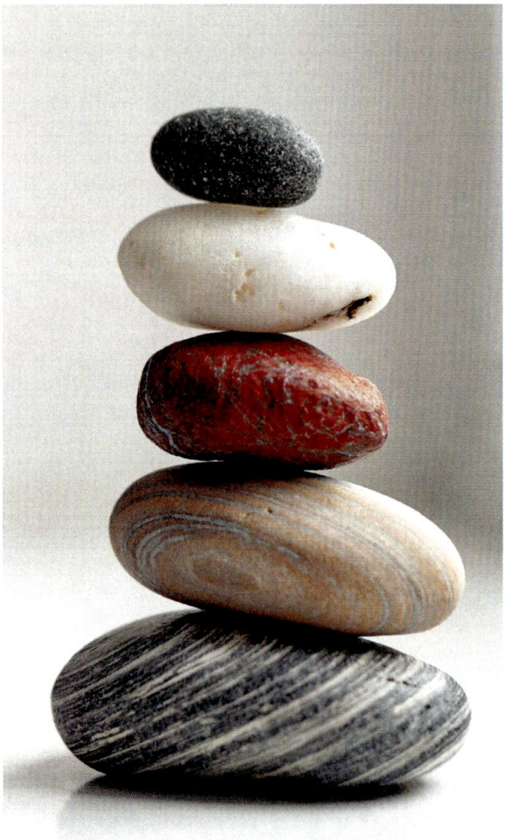

# FREEZE FAST!

**This skill is excellent when you don't want to make things worse! When you are in the moment and feel out of control just FREEZE FAST!**

FREEZE!: Don't react, don't blow your top. Freezing for a moment helps prevent you from doing what your emotions want you to do (which is to act without thinking). Stay in control and you are the boss of your emotions.

AND BREATHE: Take a big deep breath. When things are difficult it might be hard to think about what to do next on the spot. Take a step back from the situation and give yourself time to decide how to respond.

**NOTES:**

WHEN CAN I USE FREEZE FAST? (write your answer below...hint this is a great one for when you are about to get angry)

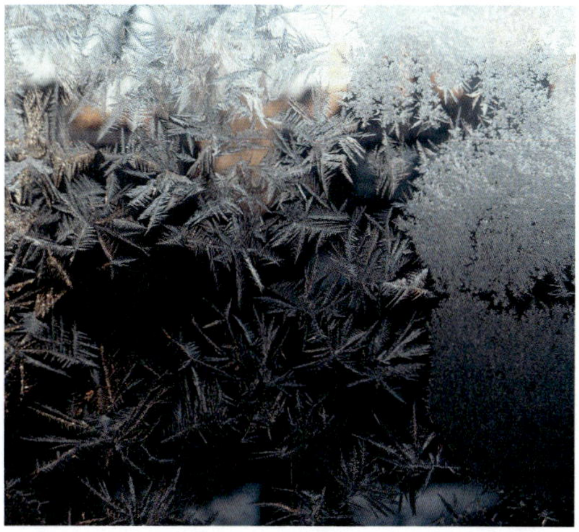

SQUEEZE; Take time to squeeze all of your muscles together at once to help ground you. This will give you time to re-group before you do the next thing!

**THINK:** Ask yourself, "What do I want from this situation?" or "What are my goals?" or "What choice might make this situation better or worse?" or "What act will allow for success?" Stay calm. Stay in control. Listen to the Automatic Negative Thoughts (ANTs) that occur...remember those are based on an outdated Belief System that was programmed into you when you were young. To make effective choices, it is important NOT to jump to conclusions. Instead, gather the relevant facts so you can understand what is going on and what options are available When you have more information and how that may impact your goals/values, you will be better prepared to deal with the situation more effectively. Remember your brain needs time to think all of this through.

# MOVE!

**This skill is intended to help you manage the emotions that you might find overwhelming. This is designed to help you quickly have some ways to get control to reduce the effects of an overwhelmed emotional mind where thinking and behaviour is controlled by extreme emotions**

**MINDFUL**: Be mindful of your reaction...Don't blow up. Watch what your body is doing and if it feels out of control then don't just stand there do something!

**OBSERVE and BREATHE**: Observe what your body is doing and just breathe. Take time to notice if you can get control of your emotions. pace your breathing by slowing it down. Breathe deeply into your belly. Slow your pace of inhaling and exhaling way down (on average, five to six breaths per minute). Breathe out more slowly than you breathe in (for example, 5 seconds in and 7 seconds out).

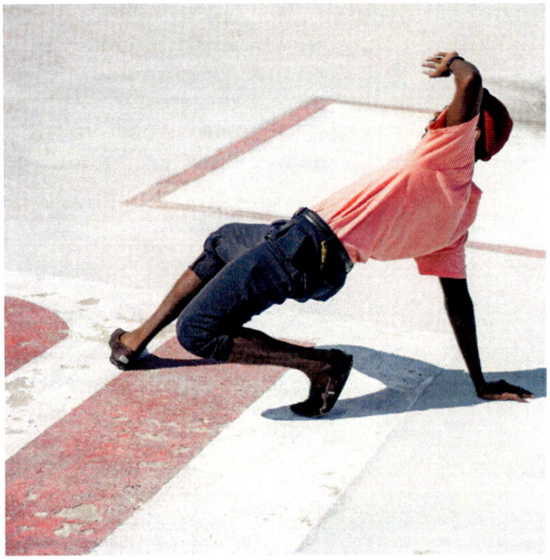

**VARY YOUR TEMPERATURE**: Use a cold Compress or ice to help you get control of your emotions. If you place a cold compress on the back of your neck or on your face you are helping send a signal to your body to relax. This activates the Mammalian Dive Reflex and our heart rate drops our breathing slows and we feel calm. By helping slow down our heart rate we reduce our oxygen consumption. This can be used to help stop a panic attack or anxiety.

**EXERCISE**: Move, move, move...move your body to regulate your emotions. Work with the reaction of your body not against...the rule of thumb is the more anxious you are the more physical you will need to be. This helps our muscles burn up excess adrenaline and helps us to regulate.........Overall this will help us to calm down so we can think more clearly.

**NOTES:**
When would I use exercise to help me manage my emotions or what are the signals in my body that tell me thigs are getting out of control? Do I feel sick in my stomach or cold?

# DROP A PIN!

**This skill is intended to help you manage the emotions that you might find overwhelming and feel like they are going to take over your entire system. It is different to Floodgates in that this is more for the moment you feel unsafe. The idea is that if you are feeling very unsafe it is giving you permission to do "something" in that moment and while we can't run away from all the difficult things that we have to endure we can also recognise that sometime we just need to do "something" that makes us feel safe...in other words we are allowed to comfort ourselves. The idea is that when you are feeling "overwhelmed in the moment" that you "drop a pin". Think of it like a map and you are doing something to feel safe in that moment. For example, if you are in a shopping centre and there are too many people around you can ask yourself "what do I need now?" and that might be a quiet place....so you go to an empty shop and it is there you can collect your thoughts.**

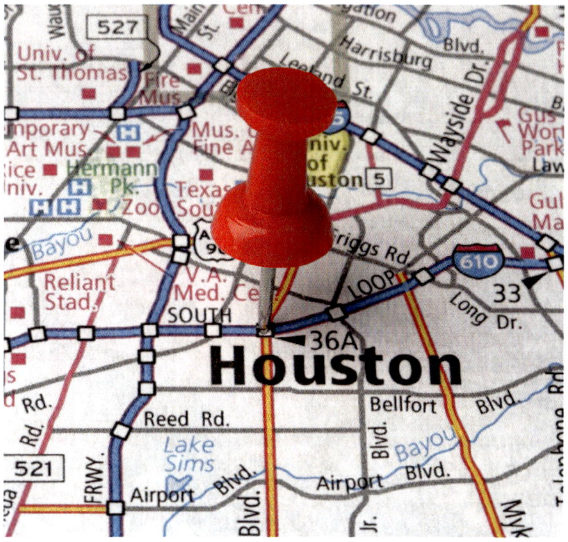


**Drop a pin:** This is a strategy for you to use when you feel "unsafe" and you need to do something in the "moment". It might be that you are in a crowded place or you are at home and your body in that moment feels "frightened or scared" and you can't think of what to do next. In a situation like this sometimes we find that we get easily overwhelmed and there is often "no particular reason" we just feel totally physically overwhelmed. This is the strategy you can use as you feel the "crisis" start so that you can do "something" and then when you are in a "safe place" physically or emotionally you can then use your crisis skills.

- As you feel your body get more and more heightened and you start to feel overwhelmed think of what you need in that moment. Ask yourself "what do I need right now!"
- Think of what in that moment would make you feel more "safe".
- Take a second to look around and then do the thing that you need to do.
- When you feel a bit "safer" you can use your crisis skills which are located in this book but a bit further on.

Example;

- If you feel "scared" but like nature, go find a tree to look at or get some fresh air.

You have already given yourself a list of safe and unsafe things on the previous pages so you already know what works for you!

# THE GLOW

**This skill is intended to help you work on a way to protect yourself from within. It is a skill that some of my clients have found very useful as they have developed a way to protect themselves from "things that upset them" by generating a protective glow. Some of my clients have used this to protect themselves from "germs" or "negativity" but others have just seen it as protective and helps them to feel safe. This skill might take a bit of work to get it to work for you and to be able to "feel" or "see" the glow when you need but over time you might find it easier and easier.**

**The Glow:** This is a strategy for you to use when you feel like you need a "protective or safe barrier" around you. This skill is one that might take you some time to become competent at while others will "get the hang" of this quickly. There is no "right" way to do this and the

colour you might choose for your "glow" can be anything that works for you. Some people have chosen a deep Emerald green and others have found that they don't need a colour to feel the "glow". Regardless, do what works for you. Once you have practiced this enough and you are confident in how the "glow" feels for you, you can summon it (hopefully) at any time you need it.

Find a quiet place and take a minute to sit quietly.

- Choose a colour that you associate with your "glow" it might be golden or it might be another colour that you associate with feeling "safe and strong".
- Sit and focus on where you think the "glow" might start from, is it your gut or is it in your chest? You could also choose a part of your body to focus on such as your hand and imagine the "glow" starting here first.
- How does the "glow" feel? What form does it take? Is it sparkling or a deep colour?
- What emotion do you associate with the "glow"? Love, joy, calm, happy?
- Sit and concentrate on the "glow" and the feeling associated with the "glow".
- Just let the feeling get stronger and stronger until you can feel it all around you.
- Notice where you feel it in particular and notice how it surrounds you.
- Now practice this until you can summon your "glow" at will.

# DO WHAT WORKS!

**This skill is intended to help you do what you need to do if have something challenging to do or something that you are needing to get through. This strategy would work particularly well if you have to have a medical procedure or treatment that you might feel scared of or that might be invasive. You don't really want to do the thing that you have to but unfortunately it has to be done. This strategy is about creating a little ritual for you to help you get through....in other words you do what works!**

**Do what works:** This is a strategy that you can use for when you have to "get through something" and whatever it is makes you feel vulnerable. Think of some things that you might need when you have to do what you need to do. Do you have a special stone or do you have a special squeeze toy? Do you need a special blanket? Do you need a special kind of cold drink, lolly or other treat? Do you have a lucky T-shirt? or lucky underwear? Crystals? Whatever it is it is ok to go and gather up these things and take them with you when you need to go to the doctor or therapist or whatever it is you need to do. Don't feel silly, these are the security blankets that you need to help you "get through". It might even be that you have a ritual? and you need to hold a squeeze ball in your hand first, look at a clock and count and breathe. Whatever it is it is ok and this strategy is giving you permission to do what you need to do. If only I had a dollar for the amount of people I know who have reported that they feel relief when their "quirks and rituals" are ok to help them get through, I could retire in the Bahamas. I know I have things that I need to do when something is difficult so rather than feel that we are odd....let's use these "rituals" that we do to our advantage.

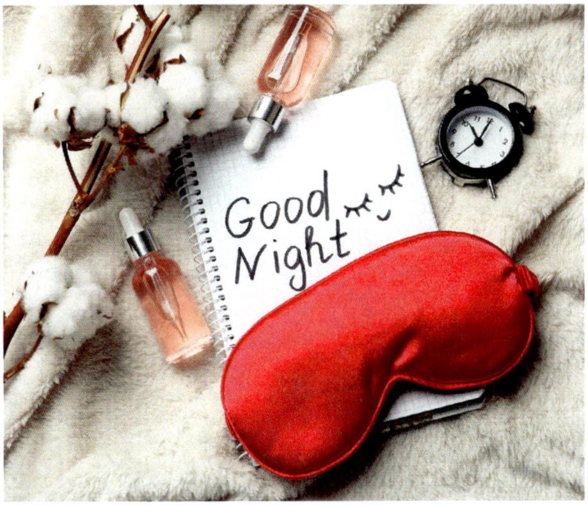


Note: we don't want the ritual to be too elaborate or involve too much stuff but rather it is discrete and works for you in the moment.

Example: While having treatment.

- Counting breathing, Squeezing a squeeze ball and thinking of the beach, while singing happy birthday in your head.
- Counting to 10 backwards, holding your breath and then make your right hand into a fist while taking a deep breath.
- Using a particular familiar smell or piece of a blanket to rub.

It doesn't matter what you need to do, just do what works!

# FLOODGATES!

**This skill is intended to help you manage the emotions that you might find overwhelming and they feel like that are going to take over your entire system. This skills is intended to teach to you to tolerate the emotion in little bites until you are more confident that you can cope. This is a skill for those of you who might struggle with thinking about emotions at all! By shutting off emotions this will help you in the short term but in the long term they are going to turn up later and be even more overwhelming than they are now. By giving yourself some time to process and feel difficult emotions as you are going through treatment you are giving yourself permission to process some of the difficult emotions along the way. The essential component of this skill is a small hard toy (most of my patients have preferred a small blue dinosaur for this exercise, so much so that KMart is constantly sold out!) to hold in your hand.**

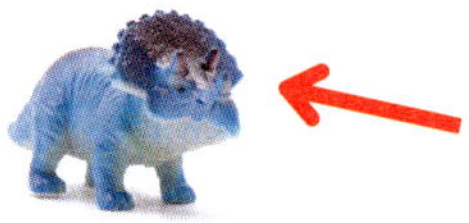

A toy just like this one but any one will do.

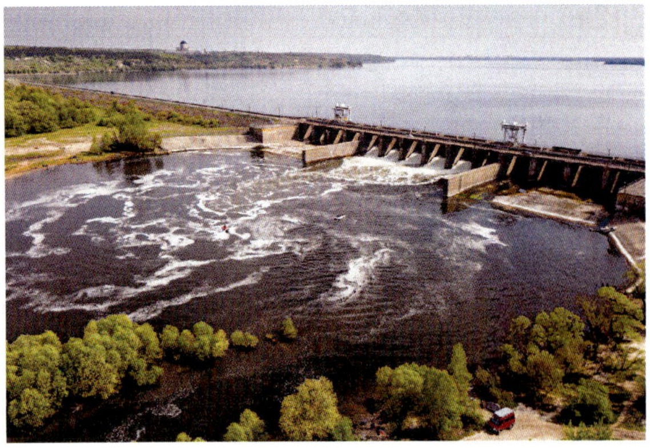

**Feel the floodgates:** Sit quietly in a place where you can give yourself a minute or two to think about your feelings and emotions. Take your small toy and put it in your hand and feel it sitting in the palm of your hand. This toy is your lifeline when the emotions are too hard or feel scary. When you feel ready just slowly turn your mind to your scary emotions. Just for a few seconds let the feelings come. Just feel the feelings. When you feel the swirl of emotions just sit with them for a few seconds and when you feel you are struggling just close your hand around the toy in your hand and squeeze it tight. You can look around the room and find something to focus on, you can even look at your hand. Now start to breathe deeply and continue to squeeze the toy in your hand. As you feel your emotions start to settle and you feel like you are slowly coming back to the room gently open your hand and give yourself time to acknowledge the emotions you have been feeling. Using this exercise you know that if you are overwhelmed by emotion you know that you have a way of re-grouping and getting control of your emotions. Over time as you practice you will get better and better at not being so scared of your emotions and you will be able to tolerate thinking about them for longer and longer periods. It is important that you understand that you have a way of not letting your emotions get out of control.

If you wanted to you could also use this when you are in pain or feeling sick from medications. Give it a go!

# DISTRACTION

People who have experienced a trauma are often distressed by memories and triggers associated with the trauma this is especially obvious when you have to have treatment and you are triggered by even the sight of a hospital. It is important that you recognise that you do not need to push these memories away all the time as- thinking about what happened is an important part of understanding what happened to you and recovering from not only the physical but also the mental aspects of treatment. However, thinking about trauma all the time can make us feel unnecessarily distressed and out of control.

Distraction techniques can be helpful for managing distressing symptoms of trauma in the moment or during times when you feel overwhelmed by intrusive thoughts, memories, or emotions. Here are some distraction techniques that can be useful and for you to consider when the negative thoughts threaten to "take over":

- **Engage in Physical Activity:** Exercise releases endorphins, which can improve mood and reduce stress.
- **Focus on the Senses:** Activities like mindful breathing, listening to calming music, a favourite scent, or holding onto a comforting object.
- **Creative Expression:** Engaging in creative activities such as drawing, painting, writing, or crafting can provide a positive outlet for emotions and thoughts related to trauma.
- **Mindfulness and Meditation:** Mindfulness practices can help individuals stay grounded in the present moment and reduce rumination on past traumatic events.
- **Distract with Activities:** Engaging in enjoyable or absorbing activities can shift attention away from distressing thoughts or emotions. This could involve reading a book, watching a movie or TV show, playing a game, solving puzzles, or cooking a meal.
- **Connect with Others:** Spending time with supportive friends, family members, or pets can provide comfort and distraction from trauma-related symptoms. Engaging in social activities or simply having a conversation with someone can help you to feel less isolated and more connected.
- **Practice Deep Breathing:** Deep breathing exercises can help calm the nervous system and reduce anxiety. Encourage slow, deep breaths in through the nose and out through the mouth, focusing on the sensation of the breath filling the lungs and the rise and fall of the chest.
- **Grounding Techniques:** Grounding techniques can help individuals stay present and connected to reality when experiencing dissociation or flashbacks. This can involve focusing on details in the environment, such as identifying objects in the room or describing textures, colours, and shapes.
- **Use Humour:** Laughter can be a powerful distraction and mood booster. Watching a funny movie, reading a humorous book, or sharing jokes with others can provide a temporary escape from distressing thoughts and emotions.
- **Practice Self-Care:** Engage in activities that promote self-care and relaxation.

Some distraction ideas!

**Count & Relax:** Breathe normally, like you might when you're just about to drop off to sleep. As you breathe in, count to yourself. As you breathe out, say "relax" to yourself. That is, when you breathe in, think "one"; as you breathe out, think "relax"; as you breathe in, think "two", as you breathe out, think "relax"; as you breathe in, think "three", and so on for ten slow breaths several times a day. Don't worry if other thoughts intrude, just gently bring your mind back to counting and breathing.

**Focus:** Focus on a small area (e.g., a square metre on the wall opposite), or on an object, and describe it in minute detail - every line, shadow, and shape. You can also use a small object to help distract you such as a small dinosaur held in your hand (remember we used this technique in Floodgates!).

**Focus on your surroundings with all your senses:** describe in detail to yourself what you can see around you, what you can hear, what you can smell, what you can feel (sensory perceptions of touch, not emotions or anxiety symptoms). Try to describe 5 things you can see, 5 you can hear, 5 you can feel, and so on. This is particularly good as it keeps you in touch with reality "here and now".

**Mental exercises:** for example, counting backwards to yourself from 1000 in 7's or naming an animal beginning with each letter of the alphabet.

Describe to yourself in great detail a happy experience from the past (e.g., a holiday, a family occasion, a favourite walk). Try to go through every aspect from start to finish. Describe in detail a place (perhaps from your past) where you feel safe, secure, relaxed, and happy.

What works? Write down the distraction strategies that help you the best when you are struggling......write down a few or add to the list when you can.

# COACHING

Self statements

It is likely that many of your thoughts are negative: worrying about the safety of yourself, concerned that you will never recover, and life will never been the same again. Mastering negative self-talk involves developing awareness of negative thought patterns, challenging them, and replacing them with more positive and realistic self-talk. Given your experience it is natural that you are fearful of the world and all the things that can happen. However, “negative self talk” can be harmful to mental well-being and can contribute to low self-esteem and increased stress. It's essential to recognize and challenge negative self-talk to promote a healthier mindset.

However if you can work out some simple things that you can say to yourself to help you calm down and relax when you are in a difficult situation or feeling overwhelmed. The best way to do this is break up tasks into manageable bite sized chunks and deal with one bit at a time.

**First**, what can I do to prepare for a situation that might be difficult for me? This helps you to re-evaluate the actual probability of the feared negative event happening - such as not being able to cope.

**Second**, What are some of the things we can say to ourselves in this situation? We can be our own coach encouraging us to get through things we want to avoid.

**Third**, managing the anxiety and distress to stop these feelings being overwhelming.

**Fourth**, This is when it is all over and you get to look back and reflect on how well you have done. This is where you get to congratulate yourself.

Examples of self-statements for coping with stress:

1. **Preparing for a stressor:**

- “What is it I have to do?”
- "I am capable and well-prepared for whatever comes my way."
- "I have faced challenges before and have come out stronger each time."
- "I trust in my abilities and skills to handle this situation successfully."
- "I am in control of my reactions and can stay calm under pressure."
- "I believe in my capacity to learn and grow from every experience."
- "I am resourceful and will find creative ways to overcome obstacles."
- "I am resilient and can bounce back from setbacks."
- "I am not defined by the outcome; I am defined by my effort and perseverance."
- "I am focused and will take one step at a time to tackle this stressor."

2. **Confronting a Stressor:**

- One step at a time; I can handle this.
- Think about what I am doing.
- The feelings I'm having are a signal for me to use my coping exercises.
- There's no need to doubt myself. I have the skills I need to get through.
- Focus on the plan. Relax ... breathe easily, I'm ready to go.
- "I will take breaks in my mind to help me cope."

- "I can prioritize and manage my time effectively. I'll focus on one task at a time and make progress."
- "I choose to focus on what I can control. Worrying about things beyond my control won't benefit me."
- "I am strong and capable. I believe in my ability to overcome challenges and emerge resilient."
- "I will ask for help when I need it. Seeking support is a sign of strength, not weakness."

3. **Coping with being overwhelmed**
- Take a breath and exhale slowly
- Focus on what is happening now, not what might happen; what is it I have to do?
- I expect my fear to rise, but I can keep it manageable. This will be over soon. I can do it.
- This fear may slow me down, but I will not be incapacitated by it.
- I may feel nauseated, but I can deal with it
- **Take a Break:** Step away from the situation, if possible. A short break can provide perspective and reduce stress.
- **Prioritize Tasks:** Make a list of tasks and prioritize them. Focus on one task at a time, starting with the most important....it might be to make an appointment you have been putting off.
- **Break It Down:** Divide large tasks into smaller, more manageable parts. Tackling smaller components can make the overall task seem less daunting. This is especially important if you are not feeling well.
- **Practice Mindfulness:** Engage in mindfulness or deep-breathing exercises.

4. **Reinforce your achievements**
- "I am proud of my achievements and the hard work I've put in to reach my goals."
- "I celebrate my successes, I am now on round three of Chemo and I am ok."
- "Doing treatment is an example of dedication, determination, and resilience."
- "I am grateful for the opportunities to have people care for me and to get well"
- "I embrace what is important to me."
- "Each accomplishment is a testament to my capabilities and the belief I have in myself."
- "I recognize and celebrate the people who are helping me."
- "I am deserving of being well and happy."
- "I attract wellness into my life, and I am open to new opportunities for growth and achievement."
- "If I can do it once I can do it again" (my personal favourite)
- "I have done a great job"

**Remember, positive affirmations are personal, and it's important to tailor them to resonate with your experiences and feelings. Regularly affirming your achievements can help foster a positive mindset and boost your confidence as you continue to pursue your goals...which is to get well.**

# CHALLENGE THE AVOIDANCE

Given that you have experienced emotional distress as part of your diagnosis it is natural that you will want to avoid and stay where it is "safe" possibly in bed with a blanket over your head. Unfortunately while that might be a nice break from reality you have some things you have to do. Over time avoiding leads to our world becoming smaller and smaller until we find that we have cut off those around us but also we have isolated ourselves from the world which makes it harder to recover or get back into life. By doing this we have also removed things from our life we used to enjoy. Cutting off things we used to like means we are more likely to become more depressed and isolated.

One idea is to challenge your "avoidance" by planning your day ahead of time and setting yourself up with things that you will enjoy or it is difficult for you to get out of, such as meeting a friend. Here are some ideas for you to consider:

Possible things to do:

- Some exercise: walk, swim, cycle ride, gym
- Some work: jobs around the house, study, chores, voluntary work
- Something for fun: a movie, museum, art gallery, window shopping
- Some social activities: visit friends, meet someone for coffee, a club or society
- Some anxiety management practice: relaxation, breathing, self-statements
- Something creative? Draw, paint?
- Walking the dog, going to a beach?
- Journaling

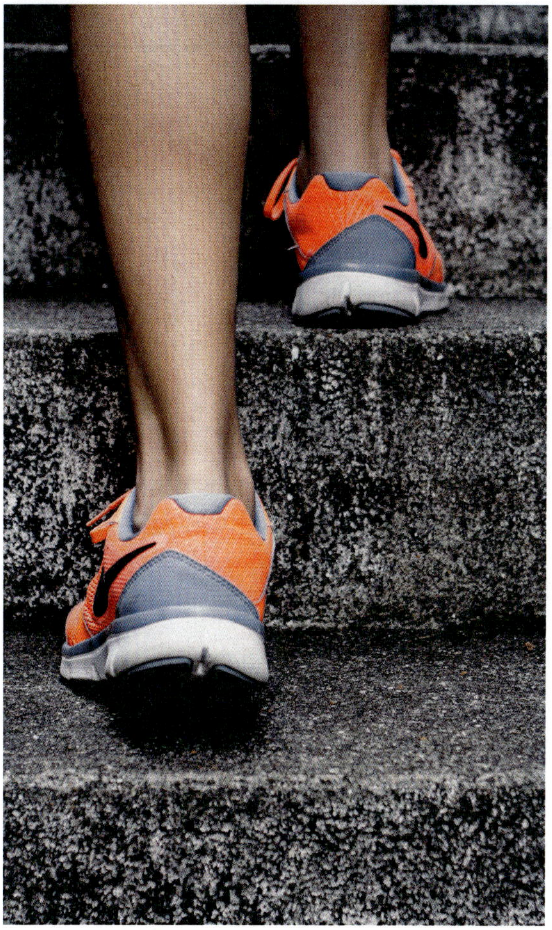

**Things I would like to do?**

# SYMPTOMS OF GRIEF

There are several stages to receiving your diagnosis and you are going to spiral through the stages of grief and trauma you are possibly going to feel all of the feelings...sometimes all at once! However, while you would like to fall apart there is simply no time. Once you are diagnosed it is a whirlwind of activity. This includes tests, being poked and prodded, tests that might be painful and worst of all telling your nearest and dearest. There is not any time to sit and avoid the whole process.

However, it is also important to remember that you are going to go through a whole pile of emotions, and that is absolutely normal. In fact there would be something wrong with you if you didn't experience emotions at a time like this. It is important to understand that while you body has betrayed you and done something to you that you had no control over, you can take control over your mind! To start with you can stop and take just a small bit of time to understand the enormity of what is going to happen or to process what is happening if you haven't already started. Mostly when we get a diagnosis that rocks our world and turns it upside down we recognise shock but we forget that there are a whole pile of other very normal emotions as well.

The stages of grief, as outlined by psychiatrist Elisabeth Kübler-Ross in her 1969 book "On Death and Dying," are often referred to as the Kübler-Ross model. However, it's important to note that grief is a complex and individual process, and not everyone experiences these stages in the same way. The stages of grief are are:

1. **Denial:** Initially, individuals may have difficulty accepting the reality of the loss. They might feel shock or numbness, and they may deny the truth of what has happened.
2. **Anger:** As the reality of the loss sets in, people may start to feel anger. This anger can be directed at themselves, at others, or even at the situation or higher powers.
3. **Bargaining:** In this stage, individuals may attempt to negotiate or bargain in an attempt to avoid the pain of the loss. They may make deals with a higher power or try to find ways to reverse or mitigate the loss.
4. **Depression:** Feelings of sadness, regret, and despair can become more prominent as individuals come to terms with the reality of the loss. This stage involves processing the emotions associated with the grief.
5. **Acceptance:** Finally, individuals reach a stage of acceptance where they come to terms with the loss and begin to integrate it into their lives. This doesn't mean they are necessarily "over" the loss, but rather that they have found a way to live with it and move forward. Acceptance takes time but when we accept a situation we can then work out ways to proactively deal with it.

It's important to recognize that not everyone goes through all of these stages, and they may not occur in a specific order. Some people may also experience stages multiple times or in cycles. Additionally, there's no set timeline for grief, and it can vary greatly from person to person. You might need some help to work thorough the grief and this is best done with professional support. There is a huge amount of loss following a diagnosis including the loss of what we knew to be normal.

Things do not have to end for us as human beings to grieve. Grief can also occur when we experience change such as the loss of a relationship, loss of a job and also when our circumstances change such as following the diagnosis and also starting treatment. A lot of things change very quickly and you are going to need time to process of the changes. These changes might not necessarily be bad things but in the short term they may feel utterly catastrophic. There are going to be limits with regards to the things that you are going to be able to do (such as getting out and going for a run, whenever you want) and also some changes in your routines. Cancer is a full time job and treatment even more so. While you may not feel and recognise grief at the time you may notice it turn up later and decide that you need to take some time to deal with it.

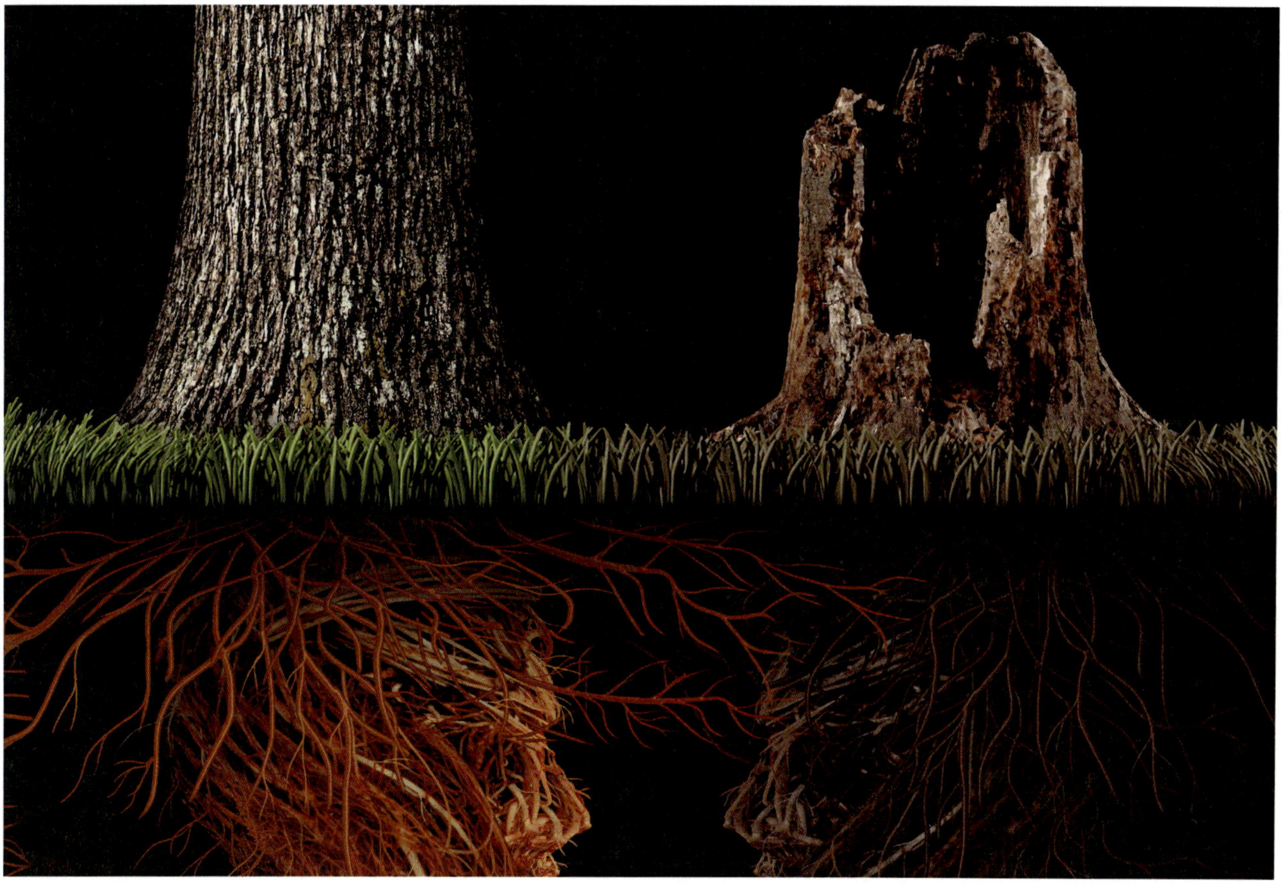

# ANGER

Anger can indeed be a significant stumbling block to recovery from cancer. While anger is a normal and natural response to a traumatic diagnosis, the way it is managed and expressed can impact the healing process. Here are some ways in which anger can hinder recovery:

1. **Increased Stress:**
    - Unmanaged anger can lead to chronic stress, which can negatively affect both physical and mental health. Prolonged stress can hinder the body's ability to recover and may exacerbate trauma-related symptoms.
2. **Social Isolation:**
    - Intense anger can lead to interpersonal difficulties, causing individuals to isolate themselves from others. This isolation can impact the support network crucial for trauma recovery.
3. **Escalation of Conflict:**
    - If anger is not effectively managed, it can lead to escalated conflicts with friends, family, or colleagues. This can further strain relationships and hinder the creation of a supportive environment.
4. **Blocking Emotional Processing:**
    - Excessive anger may serve as a defence mechanism to avoid dealing with more vulnerable emotions associated with the trauma. This can interfere with the necessary emotional processing for healing.
5. **Negative Coping Mechanisms:**
    - Some individuals may resort to negative coping mechanisms, such as substance abuse or self-harm, as a way to manage overwhelming anger. These reactions can compound trauma-related issues and seriously impact recovery. You haven't gone through all of this to make a mess now.
6. **Impact on Mental Health:**
    - Persistent anger can contribute to or exacerbate mental health conditions, such as depression or anxiety, which may obstruct overall recovery.
7. **Disruption of Cognitive Functioning:**
    - Intense anger can impair cognitive functioning, making it difficult to concentrate, make decisions, or engage in problem-solving.

To overcome anger as a stumbling block it's essential to explore healthy coping mechanisms and therapeutic interventions:

If you can recognise the warning signs of anger and intervene early, you will have a much better chance of doing something about it. Think back to the last time that you were angry and jot down a list of the first signs that appeared.

- What happened to you physically?
- What happened to your thoughts?
- What happened to your behaviour?

Once you are more aware of the triggers and the early warning signs, you will be in a much better position to use strategies or crisis skills to control your anger and not make the situation worse.

The next page has a checklist for you to work thorough regarding your anger and how you respond. Pick a time when you last got angry and try to fill in the boxes. This will help you see how you responded and how to do things differently next time. Looking at the ways you respond when you are angry is particularly important when you are frustrated by your treatment or things are not going smoothly. The last thing you want to do is "blow up" at your well meaning doctors and nurses and make it more difficult for you to have people be nice to you. Whether we like it or not if we yell at the treatment team it is going to be hard for them to feel empathy towards you and they are going to be nervous in their interactions with you. No one likes coming to work to get yelled at and that includes your doctors and nurses. Advocate for yourself....yes please do......making nurses cry....not such a great idea! Your team are human and they will be understanding but everyone has a limit.

Remember no judgement or negative self talk. Be kind to yourself.

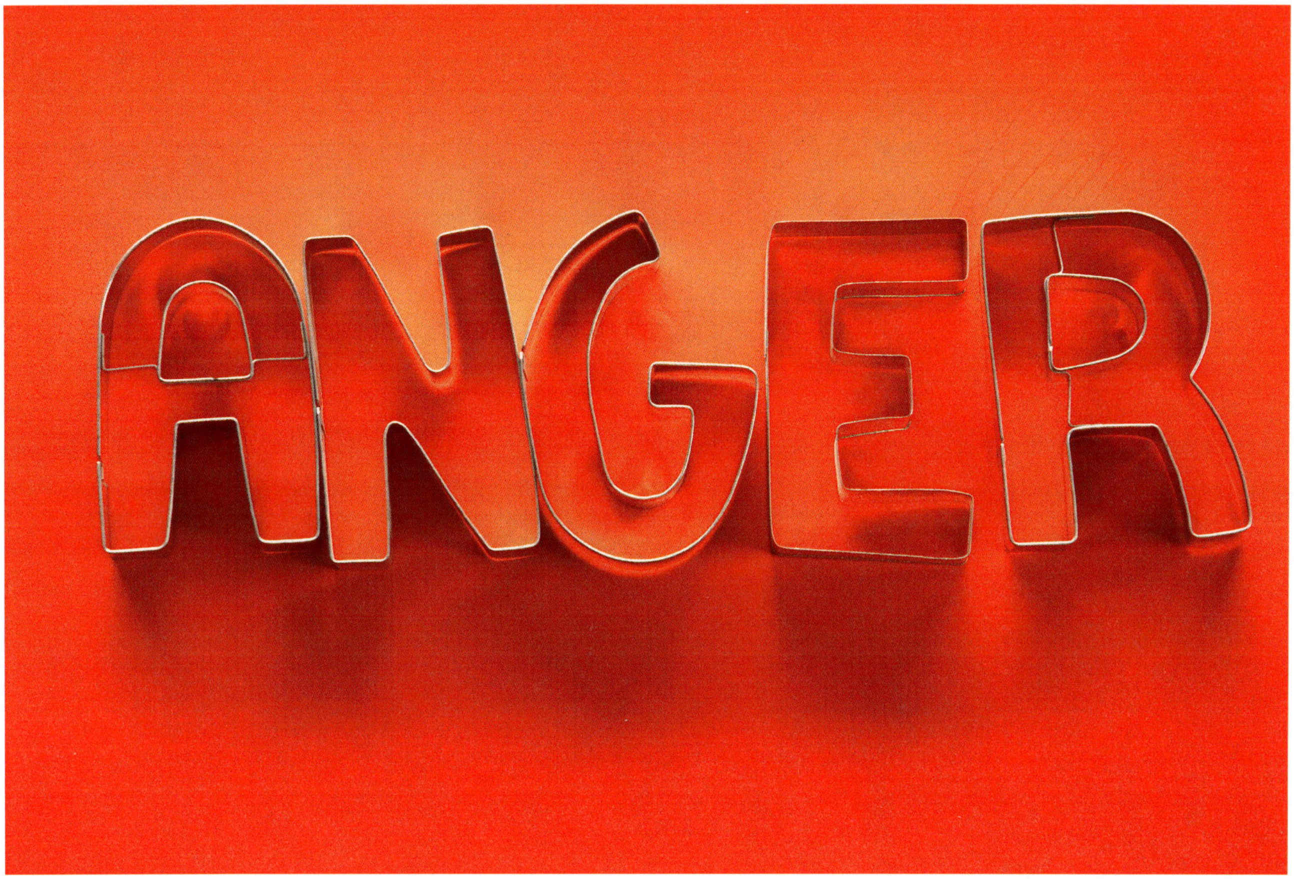

# WHAT TRIGGERS MY ANGER?

What triggered my anger? The situation

What were the thoughts? How did my body feel?

How did I react? From anger or another emotion such as fear? Did my reaction make things worse?

What strategy can I use to help me have a better response to the situation?

# OTHER EFFECTIVE STRATEGIES

Here are three additional common sense, strategies that can be very effective in managing anger:

**CONSIDER:** How do you want to be viewed if you get angry how is losing your temper going to help you? What are you really angry about? Are you in control of your anger? Will losing your temper destroy a relationship? Will you feel good about yourself if you get angry? Now consider how you want to react when angry from this headspace! What is a healthy way to act when angry? when angry from this headspace! What is a healthy way to act when angry?

**DELAY:** As we know, anger escalates very quickly so you need to find a way to stop yourself making that first angry response. Take a few slow, easy breaths and count to ten before you react. You could use the Freeze skill we talked about earlier here to help you not make the situation worse.

**TIME OUT**: If you feel the anger beginning to escalate, try to remove yourself from the situation. This does not mean storming out in a rage. It means explaining to the person you are with that you are not thinking too clearly and that you need a five minute break. Go outside or into another room and use some of the strategies described above to calm down. Then go back and try again.

**PLANNING:** Once you have identified the triggers, it is important to use that information to prepare yourself for high-risk situations. If you are going to do something that you know is likely to make you angry, choose a good moment (e.g., no other distractions, not too tired or hungry, plenty of time). Practice what you will do or say in your head beforehand.

**What have I tried ?**

**What do I like to use to help me get through my Anger?**

# COGNITIVE RESTRUCTURING

One consequence of dealing with trauma is that it may bring to the surface unhelpful thoughts and beliefs that have arisen as a result of your experiences. Aaron Beck(1963) a famous Psychiatrist called these cognitive distortions. I want to be very clear that this is totally normal! Everyone's experiences are different and your experience is unique to you and your diagnosis. It may be that you have developed an assumption from your diagnosis that you are "unsafe" or that you "won't cope". In order to recover effectively from the trauma associated with your diagnosis, it may be necessary to challenge those thoughts and beliefs (we call them "cognitions"), and try to replace them with something more rational and realistic.

Following a traumatic experience such as a cancer diagnosis, people may be left with a range of negative thoughts about what happened, and develop the view that they are very vulnerable. Similarly, sometimes people just hear the word "cancer" and just start to panic and they quite understandably fear the worst. Many people experience feelings of guilt and shame following their diagnosis thinking that somehow they did something to cause the illness. They may also have thoughts that they are "bad" or they "could have stopped it" but remember the brain is in survival mode and people often act on instinct not rational thought. People can also "beat themselves up" by thinking that they should cope better with what has happened to them and they forget they are having an extreme response to an extreme event. There is usually very little "truth" to their thoughts. Learning to challenge the thinking can help us to look at the trauma events in a more realist way. Cognitive restructuring following a diagnosis involves identifying and challenging distorted or negative thoughts and beliefs related to the diagnosis. This process is a central component of cognitive-behavioural therapy (CBT) . Here are steps you can take to engage in cognitive restructuring following trauma:

- **Identify Negative Thoughts and Beliefs**: Start by becoming aware of the negative thoughts and beliefs that you have about yourself, others, and the world as a result of the trauma. These thoughts may include feelings of guilt, shame, self-blame, helplessness, or beliefs about the world being unsafe or unpredictable.
- **Examine Evidence** : Once you've identified negative thoughts and beliefs, examine the evidence supporting or contradicting them. Ask yourself questions like: "What evidence do I have that supports this thought?" "Is there evidence that contradicts this thought?" "Am I assuming the worst-case scenario without considering other possibilities?" "Is my conclusion really likely?"
- **Challenge Distorted Thinking Patterns**: Identify common cognitive distortions such as black-and-white thinking, overgeneralization, catastrophizing, or personalization, and challenge them with more realistic and balanced thoughts. For example, if you're engaging in catastrophizing ("I'm still going to die"), challenge it by considering more realistic outcomes ("if I need to do more treatment I will").

- **Consider Alternative Perspectives**: Consider alternative perspectives or explanations for the traumatic event and its aftermath. This can involve reframing the meaning of the event, considering factors outside of your control, or acknowledging the resilience and coping strategies you've demonstrated in response to the trauma. It might mean that you value your family more as a result of Cancer.
- **Develop Adaptive Coping Statements**: Develop adaptive coping statements or affirmations to counteract negative thoughts and beliefs. These statements should be compassionate, realistic, and supportive. Examples include: "I am strong and capable of coping with difficult situations," "I am deserving of love and support," "I can learn from this experience and grow stronger."
- **Practice Mindfulness**: Use mindfulness techniques to observe your thoughts without judgment and cultivate greater self-awareness. Mindfulness can help you recognize when you're engaging in negative self-talk and create space to respond more skilfully with compassion and objectivity.
- **Gradual Exposure**: Engage in gradual exposure to trauma-related triggers or reminders while practicing cognitive restructuring techniques. This can help desensitize you to distressing thoughts and beliefs and build confidence in your ability to cope with triggers in a more adaptive way.
- **Seek Professional Support:** Consider working with a qualified therapist who specializes in working with those who have survived Cancer. A therapist can guide you through the process of cognitive restructuring in a safe and supportive environment, provide feedback and validation, and help you develop personalized coping strategies.
- **Monitor Progress:** Keep track of your progress in challenging and reframing negative thoughts and beliefs over time. Celebrate small victories and recognize improvements in your ability to cope with Cancer-related triggers and distress.
- **Be Patient and Persistent:** Remember that cognitive restructuring is a gradual process that takes time and effort. Be patient with yourself as you work through challenging thoughts and beliefs, and recognize that setbacks are a normal part of the healing journey and processing all that has happened since your diagnosis.

**By engaging in cognitive restructuring following trauma, you can gradually reduce the impact of negative thinking patterns and beliefs, increase your sense of control and empowerment, and promote healing and resilience in the aftermath of your diagnosis.**

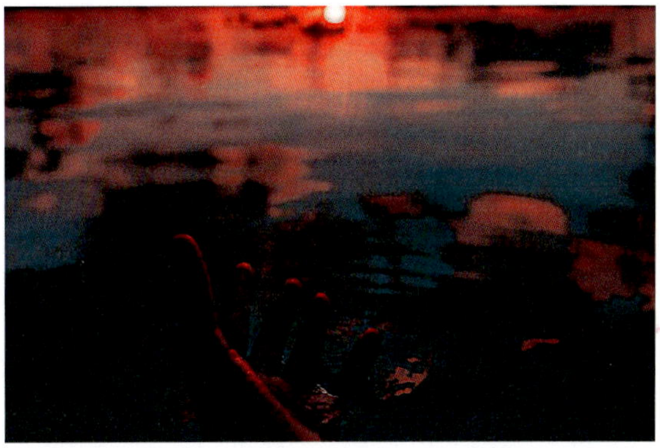

**Negative thoughts challenging exercise:**

One idea is to ask what does that emotion or thought say about me? What is the "I am statement?" For example "I am vulnerable or unsafe" or "I am unlovable". Which statement makes you feel angry? Or frightened? Or guilty? Or sad? Write this thought or belief in the section for your negative thoughts Then go through and try to see if there is any evidence for your thought. Try to identify the first time you remember the feeling this way and what were the physical feelings associated with the thought? (e.g. feel sick or anxious) What is the connection between the body, situation and brain that reinforces the negative assumption you have about yourself? Identifying these connections helps us to recognise the dysfunctional patterns in our behaviour and to see our responses to similar events is a "trauma response". We may be in a situation where we are safe and loved but our trauma response tells us the opposite. Recognising this picture is an important part of our recovery. Challenging these thoughts can help you to re-evaluate whether your thoughts and beliefs are really true.

It is normal and to be expected that you will base your assumptions around only a part of the event. Learning ways to challenge how you have interpreted the event can help identify ways to view things in a more realistic way.

TRUE
or
FALSE?

## Negative thoughts

This is not a workbook that is aimed a minimising how significant the things were that you went through. However the aim of this workbook is to find a way to have a life beyond the trauma of a Cancer diagnosis and treatment. Recovery is difficult, especially the first steps! It takes time and while you are trying to find new ways to live a different life you need to be kind to yourself and give yourself time to make mistakes and learn new ways. Life will not always be 100% safe, but try to recognise that once you find new ways to live you can start to trust and start to enjoy life again.

Most people will never understand what you went through or how scared and frightened you have been or even those dark moments you never told anyone about. With time you will learn to live a new life one that is after cancer and if cancer made you look at your life and make changes then it was not all in vain.

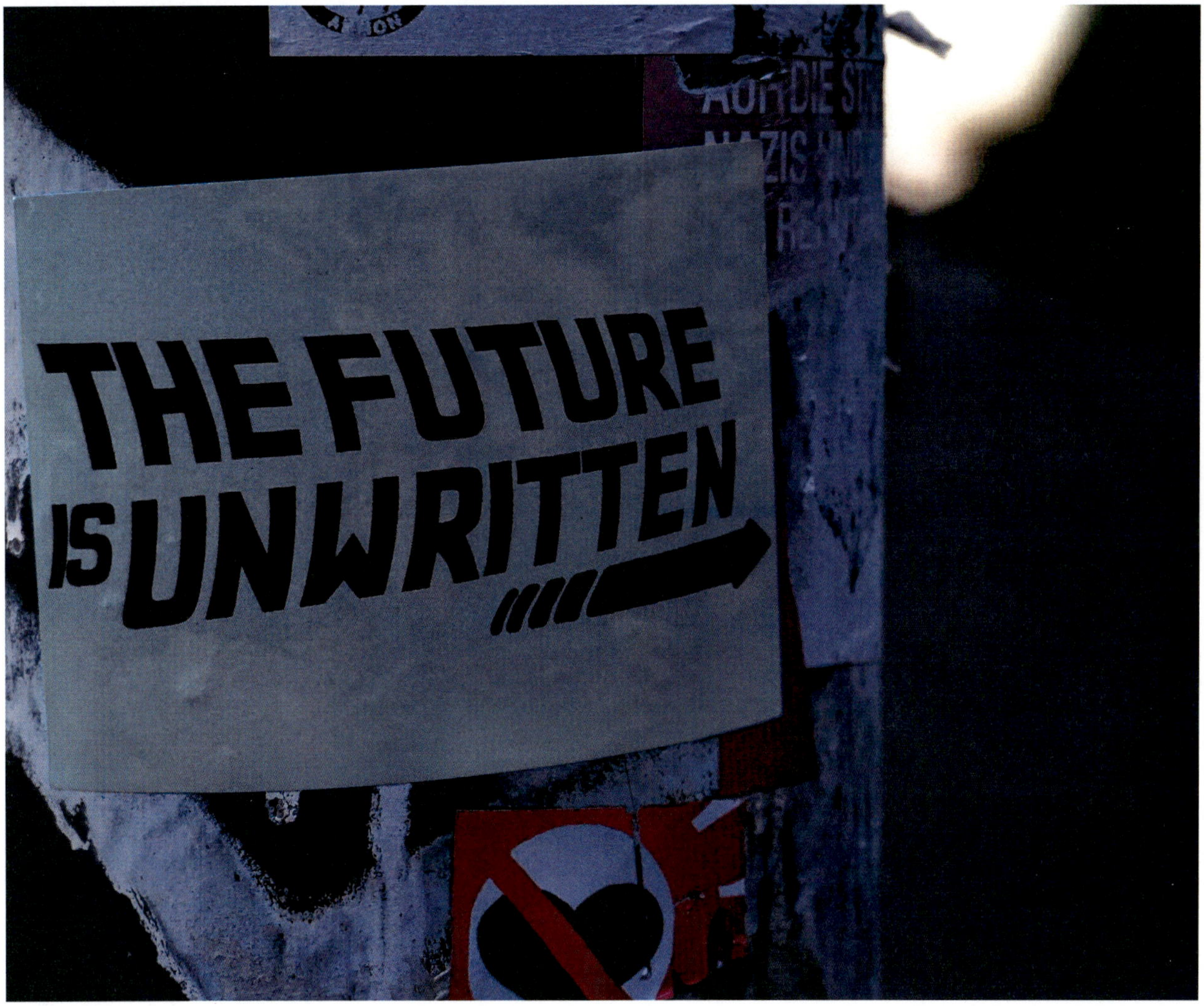

# CBT

Cognitive Behavioural Therapy (CBT) is an evidence-based approach that can be effective in addressing thought distortions that are the result of your diagnosis. We started to introduce the concept of challenging those negative thoughts in the previous section. Thought distortions, are exaggerated patterns of thinking that can contribute to emotional distress (Beck, 1963). CBT aims to identify and challenge these distortions to promote more realistic and balanced thinking. Here are some common thought distortions and how CBT can help address them:

1. **All-or-Nothing Thinking:** This involves seeing things in black and white, without considering any shades of grey. CBT can help by encouraging individuals to look for evidence of more nuanced and realistic perspectives and consider alternative possibilities.
2. **Overgeneralization:** This is when you make broad generalisations based on limited evidence or a single negative event. CBT can assist by examining the specific evidence supporting the generalisation and identifying alternative explanations or experiences that contradict it.
3. **Mental Filtering:** This distortion involves selectively focusing on negative aspects while ignoring positive ones. CBT can help by encouraging individuals to recognise and challenge this bias, actively searching for positive or neutral aspects, and considering a more balanced view.
4. **Catastrophising:** This is when you expect the worst-case scenario to happen, magnifying the potential negative outcomes of a situation. CBT can assist by examining the evidence and finding more realistic potential outcomes. Catastrophising usually shows up in our thinking as "I am going to die" even when you have the all clear! Challenging this fear is hard but try to look at the evidence. What are recurrence rates, what did the doctor say in the last visit?
5. **Personalisation:** This involves assuming excessive personal responsibility for external events or situations. CBT can help by identifying and challenging the individual's role in the event, considering other factors or people involved, and promoting a more balanced understanding of personal responsibility.
6. **Discounting the Positive:** Minimizing or dismissing positive experiences, qualities, or accomplishments. Only focusing on the negative aspects.
7. **Mind Reading:** Assuming you know what others are thinking and that their thoughts are negative or critical. A good example might be "my doctor is lying to me"
8. **Emotional Reasoning:** Believing that your feelings reflect reality. If you feel a certain way, then it must be true.
9. **Should Statements:** Setting rigid and unrealistic expectations for yourself or others. Using "should," "must," or "ought to" statements.
10. **Labelling and Mislabelling:** Attaching negative labels to yourself or others based on specific behaviours, without considering the context.

# CHALLENGING THOUGHTS

## USE THIS TO IDENTIFY AND CHALLENGE YOUR REACTION TO DIFFICULT OR CHALLENGING SITUATIONS

Situation This could be an event thought or feeling memory or image (What happened?)

| | |
|---|---|
| Initial reaction | How did I feel physically and emotionally-What did I do in the moment? (Rate intensity from 1-100) |
| Negative Automatic Thought (my unhelpful thought) | What thoughts did I notice? |
| What evidence DO I have for the thought? | See it hear it taste it touch it or smell it? |
| What evidence DON'T I have for the thought? | See it hear it taste it touch it or smell it? |
| Alternative Thought? | What is a more helpful and realistic way of thinking about this? |
| Outcome | What is a more helpful and realistic way of thinking about this? (Rate intensity from 1-100) |

# RELATIONSHIPS

Cancer can have a profound impact on relationships, affecting not only the individual diagnosed with cancer but also their family members, friends, and caregivers. Here are some ways in which cancer can impact relationships:

- **Changes in Roles and Dynamics:** Cancer can disrupt established roles and dynamics within relationships. For example, the person diagnosed with cancer may need more support and assistance from their partner or family members, leading to shifts in caregiving responsibilities and household duties. This is easy for some couples and not so easy for others. Some people find that they can happily lean on their partner and some find out that they can't. Try to speak to you partner about what your needs are and pull in other family or supports when needed.
- **Emotional Strain:** Dealing with a cancer diagnosis can evoke a wide range of emotions for both the person diagnosed and their loved ones, including fear, anxiety, sadness, anger, and uncertainty. These emotional challenges can strain relationships and make communication more difficult. This goes without saying that this will be difficult for you both and that you will both experience a wide range of emotions. If there is any issue in your relationship a cancer diagnosis is sure to bring it out in the open. Even if there were no problems before it can feel like there are issues now! It is reasonable to feel worried and to question your relationship but understand that you are both under huge amounts of strain.
- **Increased Stress and Tension:** The stress and uncertainty associated with cancer treatment and recovery can lead to increased tension and conflict in relationships. Family members and caregivers may experience heightened stress levels as they juggle caregiving responsibilities, work, and other commitments. Try to cut corners where you can and seek ways to reduce the pressure on the family. Takeaway won't hurt if it helps everyone to have a break.
- **Changes in Intimacy:** Cancer and its treatment can impact intimacy and sexual health within relationships. Physical changes, side effects of treatment, and emotional distress may affect libido, sexual function, and body image, leading to changes in intimacy and relationship dynamics. More on this in the next section under body image which might also contribute to your intimacy issues. Please remember that intimacy is important in a relationship but it also needs to be consensual. You have a right to say "no" to your partner regarding intimacy but it does not mean that you don't love and care for them. Tell them and reassure them that this is the result of treatment not a sign that things are ending in the relationship.
- **Financial Strain:** Cancer treatment and related expenses can place a significant financial burden on individuals and families. Financial worries and concerns about healthcare costs may contribute to stress and strain within relationships, particularly if there are limited resources or financial hardship. It is time to break out the savings and ensure that you use financial support where needed. If you have children in school and there are fees due, talk to the school to see what can be done to reduce pressure on the family.

- **Support and Coping Mechanisms:** Relationships can serve as important sources of support and coping during the cancer journey. Lean on those close friends and supports and also encourage your partner to do so as well, they also need support.
- **Communication Challenges:** Effective communication is essential for navigating the challenges of cancer together as a couple or family. However, communication may become more difficult due to the emotional intensity of the situation, differences in coping styles, and fear of saying the wrong thing.
- **Impact on Children:** Cancer can have a significant impact on children within the family, affecting their emotional well-being, daily routines, and sense of security. Parents may need to provide age-appropriate information and support to help children understand and cope with the cancer diagnosis and its impact on the family. Also be aware that children may need their own supports and your relationship with them is still key to them and they will need you even though you are going through treatment. Take time to listen to their concerns and validate how they feel, what their fears are and how they can work through their concerns. They are still going to want to tell you about their day and all the details of their life (young or older). Even if you put aside only a short period of time due to fatigue let your children spend time with you and help them to feel like they can still connect with you even though you are feeling tired, nauseous, or feel pain .
- **Coping and Adaptation:** Despite the challenges, many couples and families find ways to cope and adapt to the changes brought about by cancer. Give it time and try to work things out at every step of the way .

Overall, cancer can profoundly impact relationships in various ways, presenting both challenges and opportunities for growth, connection, and resilience. The important thing to remember is to not make any rash decisions or statements when you are undergoing treatment and recognise that even after treatment has finished you are still not quite yourself. Also remember that medications are going to have an impact on your thinking and now is not the time to make big decisions about the future of your relationship. Give things some time to settle and then decide if your thought process was correct or totally way off "base". I have said many times to my patients "what do you mean you think you should end the marriage?" "How about we just take 5 and think this through before you do something you might regret later, help me understand the thoughts and how you got to this conclusion".

If you are in danger or experiencing violence within a relationship please get the appropriate support and ensure that you take steps to keep you and your children or "fur" babies safe. Cancer can throw all sorts of issues into the mix and as I have said if there were issues before the diagnosis you may now have much more to deal with as you do not have the strength to tolerate another person's bad behaviour in the way that you did before. If you need to, get some help and try to work through all of the issues before making a decision. You are also going to give yourself time to regain some of your strength before you leave a relationship as you have been undergoing treatment and that is going to take a physical toll.

# ATTACHMENT

Attachment theory (Bowlby, 1969) suggests that the quality of our early relationships, particularly with primary caregivers, shapes our attachment styles and influences how we relate to others throughout our lives. When facing a cancer diagnosis, attachment patterns can influence how individuals cope with the emotional and practical challenges of the illness. Here's how attachment theory may apply to individuals with cancer:

- **Secure Attachment:** Individuals with a secure attachment style tend to have a positive view of themselves and others. They are comfortable seeking support from loved ones and are generally able to cope with stress in a healthy way. When diagnosed with cancer, securely attached individuals may lean on their support networks for emotional and practical support, which can help them navigate the challenges of treatment and recovery.
- **Anxious Attachment:** Individuals with an anxious attachment style may be overly preoccupied with relationships and fear rejection or abandonment. They may have difficulty trusting others and may seek constant reassurance and validation from loved ones. When facing a cancer diagnosis, anxiously attached individuals may experience heightened anxiety and fear about their relationships, worrying about whether their loved ones will be there for them during their illness.
- **Avoidant Attachment:** Individuals with an avoidant attachment style may be uncomfortable with emotional intimacy and may prioritize independence and self-reliance. They may have difficulty expressing their emotions and may withdraw from close relationships during times of stress. When diagnosed with cancer, avoidantly attached individuals may struggle to accept support from others and may attempt to cope with their illness on their own, which can lead to feelings of isolation and loneliness.
- **Disorganized Attachment:** Individuals with a disorganized attachment style may have experienced trauma or inconsistent caregiving in childhood, leading to confusion and ambivalence in their relationships. They may exhibit contradictory behaviours, such as seeking closeness while also pushing others away. When facing a cancer diagnosis, individuals with a disorganized attachment style may experience intense emotional distress and may struggle to cope with the uncertainty and vulnerability of their illness.

Regardless of attachment style, individuals with cancer benefit from supportive relationships and a strong social support network. Unfortunately cancer does not wait until we are in a good healthy place with all the relationships in our life before turning up...it can be at any time and if our relationship is under pressure this is only going to make things potentially much more difficult as we discussed in the previous section. Understanding our own attachment style can help us understand how we might react and how that might come across to our partner. We might push people away or reject those around us or even panic and and become very clingy. The way we cope with the diagnosis may highlight our underlying attachment style and our behaviour may suddenly become very confusing to our partner. Loved ones provide support, practical assistance and companionship during the cancer journey, hopefully helping us to feel valued, supported, and cared for during a difficult time. However, it is also expected/possible that our partner feels very helpless and confused about the way we are behaving, they may feel they can't talk to us because they don't want to upset us and push them further away.

Therapy or counselling may also be helpful for individuals struggling with attachment-related issues or coping with the emotional challenges of cancer. The opposite is also true and it may be that the diagnosis of cancer brings a couple closer together. The important thing to remember is good communication is extremely important but also trying to establish appropriate boundaries and coping skills for both partners going through this journey.

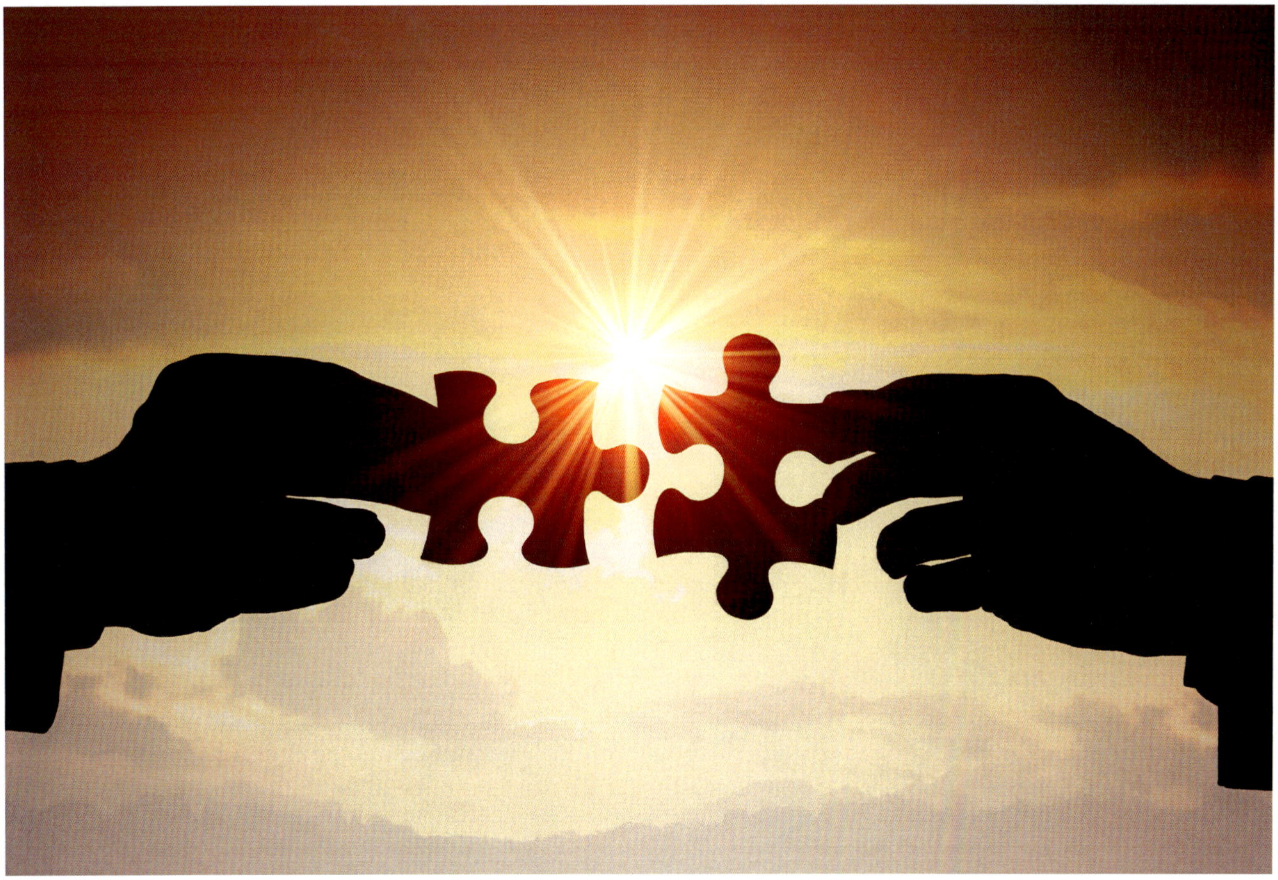

**What is a healthy relationship?**

**What is unhealthy?**

**What is my attachment style?**

**Can I say "no" in my relationship?**

# TRAUMA BONDING

Trauma bonding is commonly associated with abusive relationships, but it can also occur in non-abusive but high-intensity situations, such as during long-term cancer treatment. When a patient goes through a life-threatening illness like cancer, they may develop a deep emotional attachment to their medical team due to the dependency, vulnerability, and intense emotional experiences they share.
While this bond can be positive, providing trust, security, and support, it can also lead to emotional distress, difficulty letting go, and a sense of loss when treatment ends or changes occur (such as switching doctors or reaching remission). This is often an area of treatment that we don't discuss but it is actually very important to be aware of.

**How Trauma Bonding Develops in Cancer Care**

1. **Life-Threatening Crisis:**

- A cancer diagnosis is traumatic and creates a sense of fear, helplessness, and uncertainty. It is absolutely normal that you are terrified and that you see your doctor and the team as absolutely vital. Your team are attached to your sense of hope and survival. So while you see them as a lifeline, they are doing their job. They may not always be warm and fuzzy towards you but they care about your wellbeing otherwise they would not be working with you. This might even be more difficult to navigate if you have previous trauma in your background. After all if you have had people betray you in the past it is going to be difficult for you to trust as part of your treatment. Regardless it is very normal for you to become very invested in your doctor and medical team and want them to think well of you and for them to want to help you to recover. You are very vulnerable and this is normal but remember that while you see them as a lifeline they are there to do a job.

2. **Dependence on Medical Staff:**

- Patients rely on doctors, nurses, and caregivers for both physical and emotional support. As I have already stated this is normal but your doctor is a Cancer Specialist and not a therapist. However it is important to understand that they have good and bad days and if they are a bit "off" it is ok, they are not going to drop the ball. They are human too and they have to stay focussed on the end goal...getting you better.
- Trusting them with life-or-death decisions strengthens the emotional bond which makes absolute sense and you are putting your life in their hands. While they know (just about) everything about you they still need to maintain boundaries to be able to be objective about your care. If you feel like you are not getting your needs met you might need to speak to someone about this to try and get some perspective.

3. **Emotional Highs and Lows:**

- The cycle of bad news (test results, setbacks) and good news (remission, successful treatments) mirrors the push-pull dynamic seen in trauma bonding. Let's face it the big C is all about the highs and lows. It is all about what it going to happen next and also through all of this you are reliant on them to help you through to the other side. It is helpful to know that the push and pull with regards to your treatment is very similar to the way people trauma bond in a bad relationship. Ironic isn't it, that you are reliant on someone to help you cope and get well and they are also the bearer at times of bad news and yet you can still be happy to see them as you see them as a very definite part of your world. Your children will know who they are, your friends and family and they can feel like an old friend. This is important as you need to be able to trust your doctor but understand the bond for what it is which is they care for you but they will have to at times maintain boundaries and if they do it can make us worry that something is wrong. Often there is nothing wrong but they need to do their job.

- Patients can feel emotionally tethered to their medical team and while this is important they will know more about us than we know about them. This is where boundaries come in and a good team will support you but also maintain boundaries with you.

4. **Intimate & Vulnerable Moments:**

- Cancer treatment often involves physical and emotional exposure (surgeries, chemotherapy, discussing fears of death, body changes, etc.). The medical team sees the patient at their most vulnerable, deepening attachment and there is going to possibly be a lot of intimate moments with your doctors and team. The important thing is to understand why you are attached to these people and it is due to treatment not because you have met them at the pub or in the school yard and you would have chosen to be their friend. In fact if you did get to know them outside of your treatment you may have absolutely nothing in common. However while going through treatment they can feel like your best friend and you can feel like you are part of the gang. This is important but also recognise that it is not permanent and that is why it is so important to maintain your friendships as these people will be there for your when this is over.

5. **Intermittent Reassurance & Comfort:**

- The medical team provides reassurance, empathy, and support through painful experiences. The patient may begin to equate their emotional safety and survival with the presence of their doctors and nurses. and this is difficult when you are really struggling. Remember at the start of this book we talked about your crew? While the doctors and medical team are hopefully trauma informed and can help you in the right way when you need them too they are not trained counsellors. It is vital if you are struggling to get a counsellor to help you. The great thing about a counsellor is that once this is over they can still be there to support you and to help you to manage all of the feelings that you have about your cancer and treatment team all the highs and lows and strategies to help you get through to the other side.

6. **Fear of Abandonment (End of Treatment or Doctor Changes):**

- When treatment ends or a doctor retires, the loss can feel devastating, triggering grief, anxiety, and even identity confusion ("Who am I without my cancer team?"). This mirrors the loss felt in trauma bonds, even though the relationship was professional, not personal. This is absolutely a big one!!! Especially if you need to see your doctor for "check ups" every few months or every year. If this is the person who helped you get to the "other side" then you are naturally going to feel very attached to them. Normal all normal!! However, they have lives too and yes one of these days they will tell you they are retiring or moving on. It is normal for you to recognise that you are going to be upset and possibly even devastated. Further they may transfer your care to another clinician and team and you may not like them to start with or have no faith that they know what they are doing. After all they are not Doctor Such and Such who is 65 years old and a bit rough around the edges but he really knew what he was doing. Now you are in a position where you have to get to know the "new one" who is only 42 and looks about the same age as your son! It is normal that it is going to take some time to adjust but just remember that you can't just call yourself a Medical Doctor without some pretty serious qualifications. Further, your doctor would not transfer you to just anyone as they are invested in your well being.

  If you find yourself in the very difficult position of not liking your new doctor or you do not have faith in them then we have a problem. In this case let's dust off those advocacy plans we spoke about earlier in the book and it is time for you to be an advocate for yourself and to find someone you do trust and can try to build a working relationship with. We can't like everyone but it is very important that you trust your team and feel that they are invested in your ongoing care.

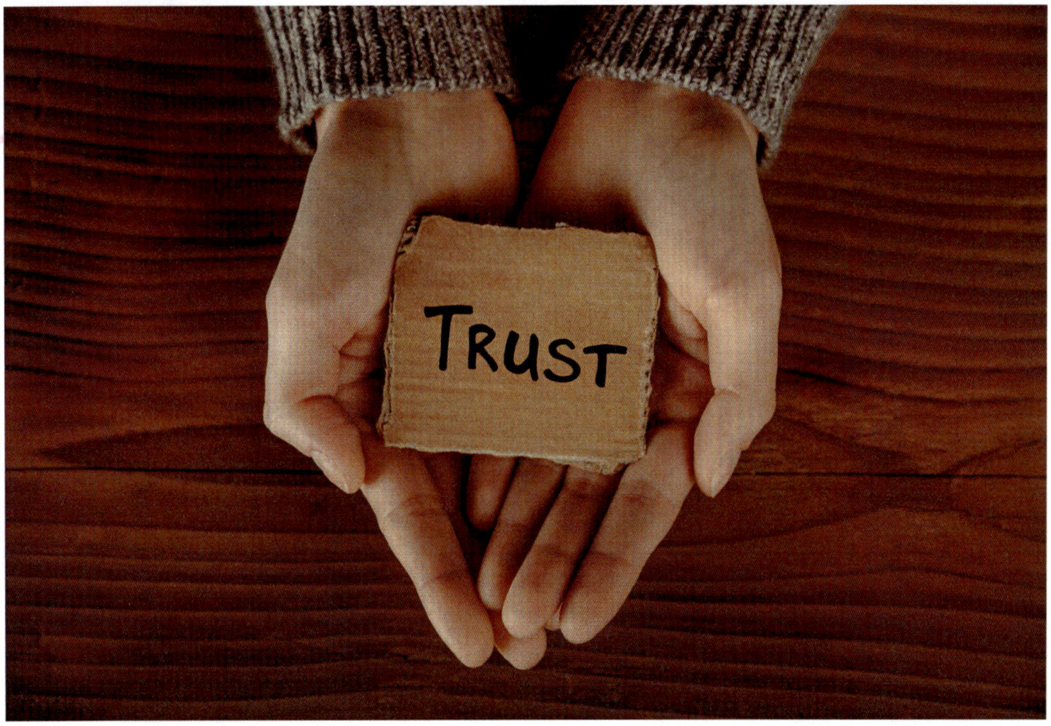

# SIGNS OF TRAUMA BONDING

Signs You May Be Experiencing Trauma Bonding with Your Medical Team

- Feeling anxious or lost at the idea of finishing treatment or switching doctors.
- Believing that only this specific medical team can care for you properly.
- Feeling a deep emotional attachment to your doctors or nurses beyond medical care.
- Struggling with a sense of abandonment or grief when treatment ends.
- Avoiding independence and struggling with post-treatment transitions.
- Feeling resentful, betrayed, or panicked when a doctor is unavailable.
- Difficulty trusting new healthcare providers.

If you ticked most of these boxes it is great that you have recognised that this might be an issue for you. If your trauma bonding is unhealthy with your team it can perhaps get in the way of your care and might make it hard for your team to maintain boundaries, especially if you are pushing them and if you are overly reliant on them emotionally. In this sort of situation please talk to someone about the issues and how they can be resolved so that your team can do what they do best and you are able to get the support you need.

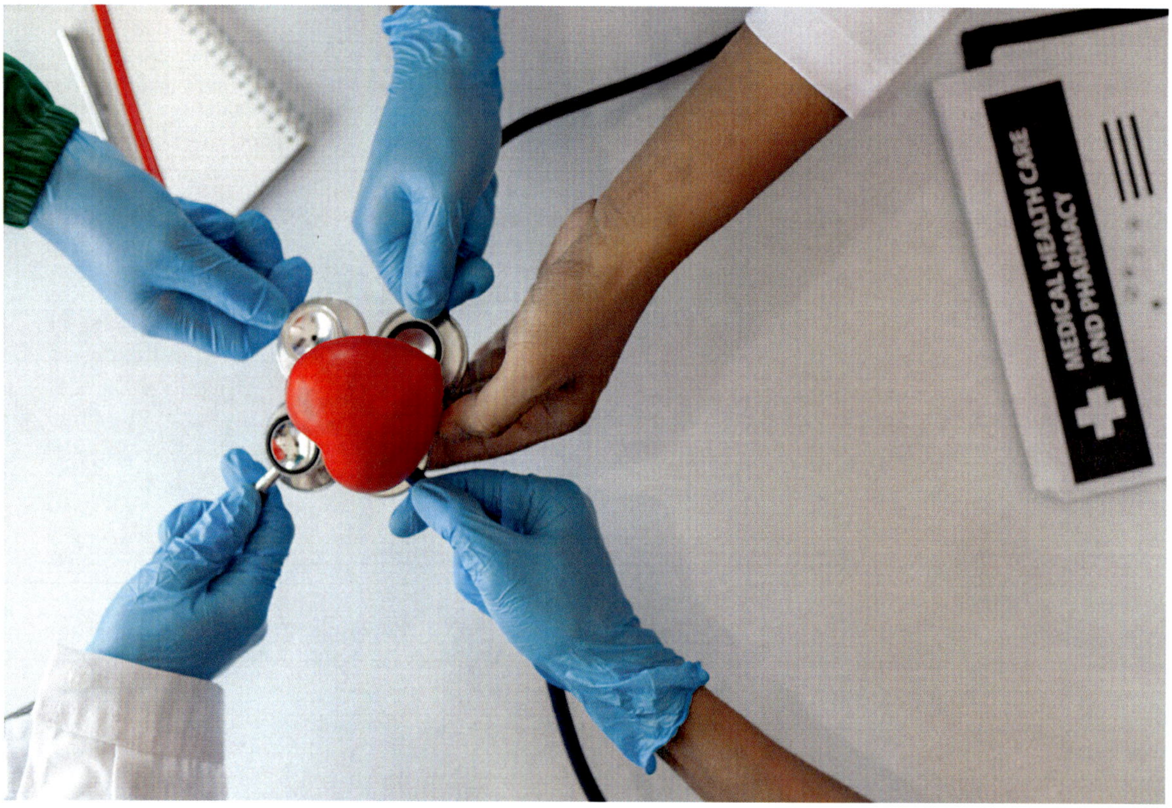

# NAVIGATING THE BOND

Navigating the Emotional Challenges of Trauma Bonding in Cancer Care

🖤 1. **Recognize & Acknowledge the Bond:**

- It's natural to feel attached to those who helped you through a life-altering illness. Acknowledge that this bond is a response to trauma, not a weakness. It is very normal but it is a sign that you might need some extra support and help navigating your emotions. The important thing is that you recognise the connection for what it is and not try to make more of it than it is. Seek out support and also connect with your friends or others who can relate.

🖤 **2. Process the Fear of Letting Go:**

- The end of active treatment can feel like a loss of safety. While it has been obviously very difficult it is reassuring to go to the same place on a routine basis and feel secure that you are doing treatment. After such an intense time suddenly not doing treatment is going to feel very weird and also frightening. Just because you don't like something doesn't mean you won't miss it when it is gone.
- Work through post-treatment anxiety and uncertainty with therapy, journaling, or support groups. Seek help and recognise that it is ok to feel worried. Acknowledging the feeling is the first steps to working out what you are going to do about it.

🖤 3. **Shift Perspective: You Are Your Own Healer:**

- Your medical team was a guide, but your strength carried you through. Regardless of what happened at the end of the day you were the one who kept turning up to treatment and who did what you needed to do. You can own that and feel confident that if you continue to trust yourself you will know what to do next.
- Recognizing your own resilience helps reduce dependency.

🖤 4. **Seek Emotional Support Elsewhere:**

- Transition emotional support from your medical team to trusted friends, family, therapists, or survivor groups. There are probably already a lot of people about who you have been leaning on or people you have been able to talk to. Go and seek these people out and see if they felt the same way you did.
- If you struggle with post-treatment emotions, consider therapy with a cancer-informed counsellor. We have spoken about this before and it is important to recognise the importance of this to help you manage things if you feel like you are struggling.

🖤 5. **Create a New Support Network:**

- Build connections outside the hospital (mentors, survivor networks, hobbies, community groups). Try to connect with others who have gone through what you have gone through (just make sure the group is healthy and you are comfortable). It can be very reassuring that others will say the things that you thought you were the only one who felt that way.
- Engaging in life beyond cancer can help lessen dependency on the medical team

🖤 6. **Allow Yourself to Grieve the Transition:**

- Finishing treatment or losing a trusted provider can feel like a breakup or a major life transition and it is exactly that. Your team have been part of a very intense time in your life and you need to give yourself time to feel the loss. One day all of these people have been around you and now suddenly they are gone. It is a bit like being kicked out of the gang. Adjusting might take some time and it is normal to feel like you are missing out or grieving these people. Believe me though when I say this as a therapist I love it when people drop me a line to tell me how life has progressed for them but I am never so delighted as when people tell me that they don't want to see me anymore as they don't need me. That is kind of the point after all.
- Give yourself time and space to grieve while also embracing new beginnings.

🖤 7. **Focus on Meaning & Growth:**

- Shift the focus from holding on to the past to moving forward with purpose.
- Explore new passions, volunteer work, or advocacy for other patients.

Trauma bonding with a medical team is a real emotional response to the intense experience of battling cancer. While it reflects trust, appreciation, and the deep impact of compassionate care, it can also lead to fear, anxiety, and loss when the relationship changes or ends. Recognizing this bond, processing emotions, and gradually shifting support to friends, family, and survivor networks can help patients transition from survival mode to thriving.

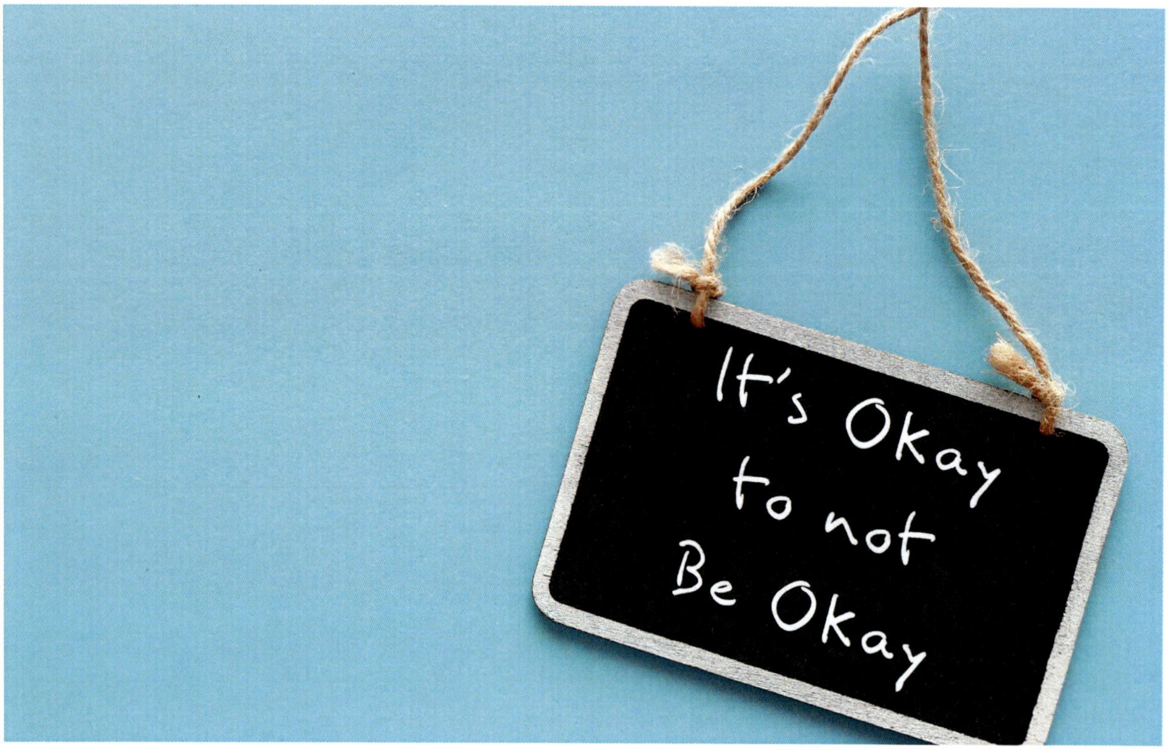

# BODY IMAGE

Cancer and its treatment can have a significant impact on body image, which refers to how individuals perceive, feel about, and relate to their bodies, which is obvious. Here are some ways in which cancer can affect body image:

- **Physical Changes:** Cancer treatment, such as surgery, chemotherapy, radiation therapy, and hormone therapy, can cause visible physical changes to the body. These changes may include hair loss, scars, weight fluctuations, changes in skin tone or texture, loss of muscle mass, and changes in body shape or appearance. Lots of people might tell you that nothing will change but that isn't so and while they mean well it is setting you up for possibly unrealistic expectations. Even after treatment and even if everything has gone well it still might take time for everything to settle and for you to start to look more normal and like yourself.
- **Surgical Scars:** Surgery is a common treatment for many types of cancer, and surgical procedures may leave visible scars on the body. Scars can affect body image by altering the appearance of the skin and reminding individuals of their cancer diagnosis and treatment experience. Some people can become very distressed by the scars as a result of treatment and others choose to see them as "battle scars" or "spoils of war" and take pride in them.
- **Hair Loss:** Chemotherapy and radiation therapy can cause hair loss or thinning, which can have a profound impact on self-esteem and body image. Hair loss may not only occur on the scalp but also eyebrows, eyelashes, and body hair, leading to changes in appearance and self-perception. However not everyone loses their hair. When a friend started to lose her hair she decided to get it shaved and frankly it really suited her. Together we also found a whole pile of cool head covers which she really liked. Some people decide that they want to try a wig and the quality of the wig can certainly make a difference to whether or not you will want to wear one. Wigs can be made out of a variety of materials but have a play and see if you are comfortable or want to wear one. You might decide that you preferer to go natural! This is a huge issue for some people (losing your hair) and can be a real point of trauma for them. Also when your hair grows back after treatment it might be different which can be just as much of a challenge and readjustment.
- **Changes in Sexual Function:** Cancer and its treatment can affect sexual function and intimacy, leading to changes in libido, arousal, and sexual satisfaction. Physical changes, such as fatigue, pain, hormonal changes, and body image concerns, may contribute to sexual difficulties and impact relationships. When you think about it, it is not surprising. You are going to be struggling just to do the basics and your libido might just be non-existent! This is very hard for couples who prior to the cancer diagnosis had a very active sex life. Suddenly not wanting to have intimacy in the relationship can feel like a rejection for your partner. Just remember it is not permanent and hopefully things can get back on track in the future but for right now there are going to perhaps be times you just don't want to "do it". Also sometimes after cancer it is very difficult to re-engage intimacy with your partner.

There can be a number of different physical reasons struggling to regain intimacy or it might be a sign of something else going on in the relationship.

- **Body Confidence:** Cancer treatment can challenge individuals' sense of body confidence and self-esteem, leading to feelings of insecurity, self-consciousness, and inadequacy. Changes in appearance or physical abilities may make individuals feel less confident or comfortable in their bodies. It is **normal** after invasive treatment to not feel as strong or as confident in you body as you did before. Further, depending on how you have responded to treatment and also the treatment you have you may still have some after effects such as sensitivity in hands or feet. We are all different and respond differently to treatment. The important thing to remember is that you have just run a "marathon". While it might be a bit disconcerting that your "face id" on your phone isn't recognising you due to a puffy face from steroids or that your clothes don't fit the way they did pre cancer give yourself some time to find out how things settle.
- **Functional Impairments:** Cancer and its treatment may result in functional impairments or limitations that affect daily activities and quality of life. Physical symptoms such as pain, fatigue, weakness, or mobility issues can impact individuals' ability to engage in activities they enjoy and affect their body image. Again...you have just run a marathon and you are going to take some time to build up your strength. There is plenty of evidence to suggest that if you exercise during your treatment that you are gong to cope better in the long run but you have to be realistic and take it easy and grow your strength and fitness over time. It might take a while but perhaps get some support from an exercise physiologist or personal trainer who specialises in the area of those recovering from cancer who can organise you a fitness program.
- **Psychological Impact:** Body image concerns related to cancer can contribute to psychological distress, anxiety, depression, and poor quality of life. Negative body image may interfere with social interactions, relationships, and overall well-being, leading to feelings of isolation or withdrawal. It can be very difficult for people to accept the emotional distress they may feel after going through treatment especially if they have never had mental health problems prior to their diagnosis. Unfortunately psychological issues have a way of creeping up on us and it might be advisable if you are finding that you are struggling to seek out an appropriate therapist who works with body image concerns and cancer. At times when we are struggling psychologically we don't realise the impact our mental health is having on those around us. We might take out our frustrations on our family or those who are important to us. It is important to remember that they have gone through this journey with you and while they recognise the distress you might be feeling they are possibly also struggling with the changes in your body and reduced physical capacity. Acceptance of the physical changes is very difficult especially if you are still undergoing treatment and unsure how things are going to end up in the long run. It is surprising how many people end up discussing this issue in therapy but it's not one that we often talk about publicly. A friend stated that she felt guilty for

talking about the changes in her body after cancer as everyone assumed that she should be "grateful" for being in remission. As the same friend also pointed out to me she **was** grateful for being in remission but she had never **asked** for cancer in the first place and adjusting to the changes in her body was not something she wanted to have to deal with having been fit and healthy all of her life. Generally she was "pissed off" that she had done all of the "right things" (not smoke and drink) and then she got cancer and now her body was "weak" and she struggled to open a jar of "pickles". Not fair! She of course had a right to be angry, and no it wasn't fair.

- **Social Stigma:** Cancer-related changes in appearance or physical function may be associated with social stigma, stereotypes, and misconceptions. There are lots of new advances which allow treatment to go "with us" if we go out into public. We are also going to look different to people who have seen us in one setting (with our hair looking healthy) and these same people are potentially going to be a little confronted or unsure if they see us looking different. This might be further complicated if we are carrying Chemo medication around our neck, especially if it is a bright red colour which makes it hard to hide. If you are going to go out in public take people with you who might be supportive or go to places that you feel comfortable. Familiar places will help you to be more at ease and hopefully once people see you a few times they stop reacting differently. You have a right to go out in public and it will be good for you to feel like you are part of the world again. There may be times however when you are immunocompromised and may need to wear a mask or distance a bit physically from people. Fortunately we have a lot to thank COVID for and you are more likely to get away with this now than prior to COVID when masks were much less frequently used or accepted in public. You have every right to go out in public and you have nothing to be ashamed of. You have been dealing with one of the most difficult things possible and you have nothing to be embarrassed about. Besides people who judge you have no idea what their future holds and might be grateful to remember how you coped when they saw you in public. Their reaction might also indicate they have their own issues to deal with.
- **Coping Strategies:** Coping with changes in body image related to cancer involves developing adaptive coping strategies and self-care practices. This may include engaging in relaxation techniques, practicing self-compassion, and focusing on aspects of oneself beyond physical appearance. It might be that you have to get some help regarding this and starting to think about who you are besides the cancer diagnosis. We focus a lot on the way we look and it can be very upsetting when we feel we don't look normal or the way we did before the diagnosis. Being able to reframe that we are not only about the way we look but that we have lots of other qualities that are important might be a way to help you accept that there is more to you then your outward appearance. Please don't get me wrong, it is expected that you are going to find it very confronting and it's not as simple as "snapping" your fingers and changing the way you think. There are going to be strategies that are going to help particularly as there is nothing you can do about your situation but once you accept it you can find ways to help you cope better with it.

- **Reconstructive Options:** Individuals who experience significant changes in body image due to cancer treatment, may decide to look at reconstructive surgery or cosmetic procedures to restore physical appearance and improve self-esteem. These procedures can help individuals feel more comfortable and confident after cancer treatment. For example, some people who have had breast cancer get surgical reconstruction if they have had a mastectomy. Additionally it may have been that you have had skin cancers in a prominent place that were removed leaving a scar. It is worth investigating your options and also if you are eligible for private health or Medicare rebates for reconstructive surgery. Surgery after cancer is a very private choice and it is one that should be carefully considered with medical advice and you should not feel pressured to do something that you are uncomfortable with.

Overall, cancer can profoundly impact body image, affecting individuals' perceptions, feelings, and relationships with their bodies. By acknowledging and addressing body image concerns, individuals can take steps to cope with changes, cultivate self-acceptance, and focus on aspects of themselves that go beyond physical appearance.

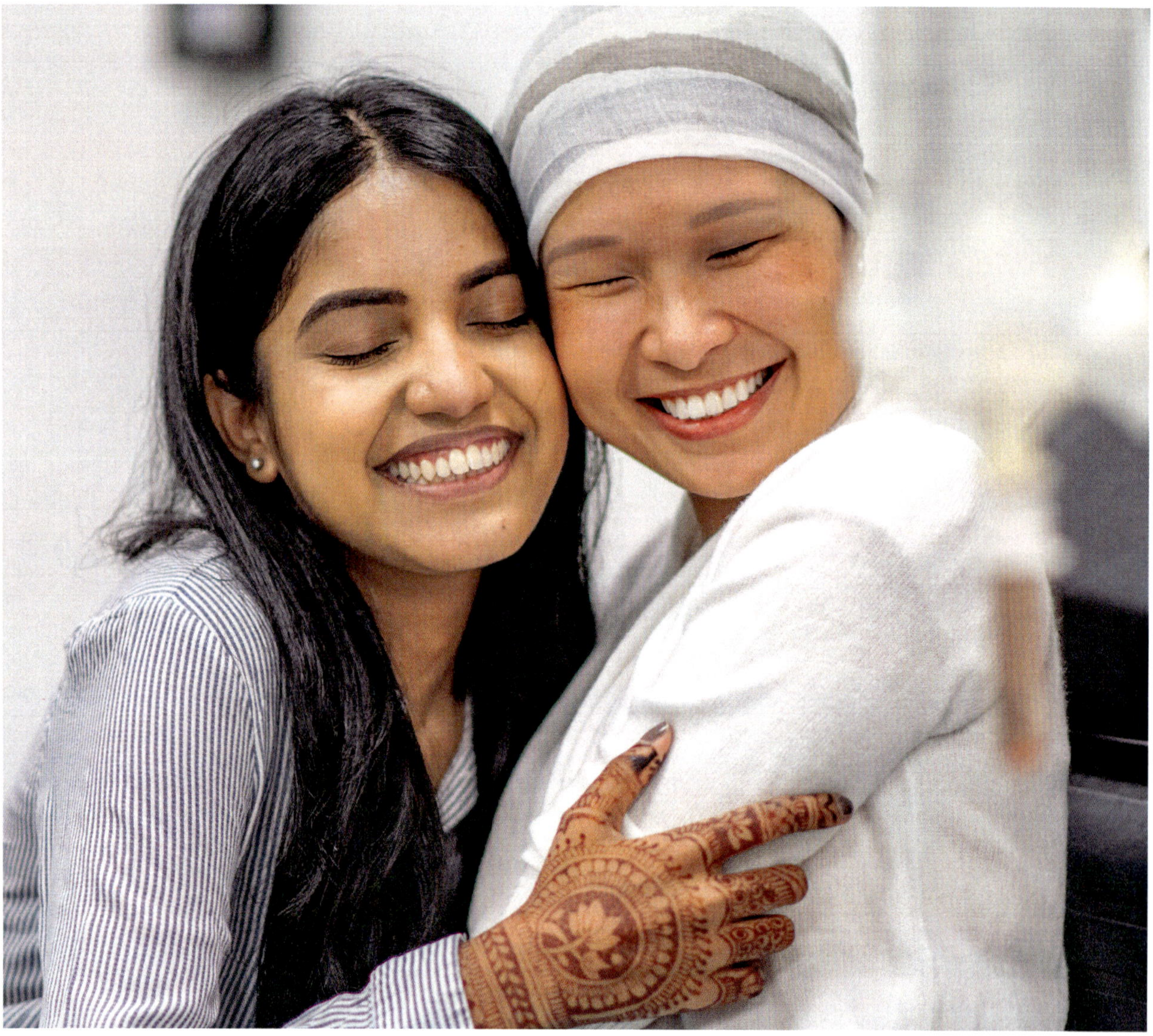

# FEAR OF RECURRENCE

Okay so now you have done the treatment and the doctor has told you you are in the clear. You are now in the process of starting to put you life back together and understand all of the things that have happened to you over this period of time from point of diagnosis through to treatment. The dust is just starting to "settle" and you feel like everything is just starting to come back to earth. However there is still the fear. The fear of cancer recurrence is a common experience for many cancer survivors. Even after successful treatment and being declared cancer-free, the fear of the cancer returning can persist and have a significant impact on one's emotional well-being and quality of life. The fear is **normal**. Here are some key points about the fear of cancer recurrence:

1. **Normal Response:** It's important to recognize that fear of cancer recurrence is a normal and understandable response to having faced a life-threatening illness. The experience of cancer can shatter one's sense of security and trust in their body, leading to ongoing anxiety and worry about the possibility of the cancer returning. In this book I have used the word **normal** a number of times but let's face it there is nothing normal about being faced with a life-threatening illness, the invasive treatment that comes with that and then the not having any guarantees or knowing that the cancer won't return. I would love to give you a magic wand and wave my hand about and give you a guarantee but the reality is that that is not possible. Hopefully your doctors have spoken with you about the outcomes and I think it is very important to acknowledge that they do this every day for a living, they are trained and are specialised in the area. However even they can't give us 100% guarantee. In some ways this is a leap of faith and recognising that we might choose to live life differently compared to prior to the diagnosis. In some ways it can feel like you are living on the edge of an abyss and you are unsure of what is next. Recognise that it might take time for you to accept this and also those around you to accept there are no guarantees of recurrence. It might also feel like you are waiting for the next bomb to drop but it is important to try and learn to live with all that is happened to you rather than live in fear. Fear isn't going to help you it is only going to stop you doing things and living life to the best of your ability.

   Radical acceptance can help us with this where we are accepting that we don't have to like something but we have to accept the situation. Once we can accept the situation we are able to find solutions to the problem and challenge our fears and anxiety. For example if we have a fear of recurrence we might be so scared that we don't spend time with people we care about but that is only going to isolate us and there is no evidence that we are ill today. Challenging the things that you are frightened of and looking at the evidence and facts is a good way to help you slowly accept that fear is normal. Further, this will also help you recognise that you have survived! You are here! You get to now enjoy and spend time doing things today that a few months ago were possibly very out of reach. One friend said to me "I now get to wear the nice clothes, eat the nice food drink the wine and spend time with my children".

2. **Triggers:** Various factors can trigger or exacerbate the fear of cancer recurrence, including routine follow-up appointments, medical tests or scans, anniversaries of diagnosis or treatment milestones. Experiencing physical symptoms that may be unrelated to cancer but trigger anxiety, and hearing about others' experiences of cancer recurrence can also trigger distress. Lumps and bumps is additionally potentially going to be frightening and have you rushing back to the doctor. It is natural that pains and weird symptoms might have your anxiety escalating. While it is important to not ignore symptoms that are unusual and seek medical advice if this is the case it is also advisable that you recognise you are going to be much more hypervigilant and anxious to all of your physical symptoms compared to prior to your diagnosis. If there is something that you are really concerned about please seek medical advice. Alternatively another good way to try and settle your anxiety is to use the **five rule**. The **five rule** is think of five symptoms that are connected to your anxiety such as if you have a fear of your cancer returning what are five symptoms that may indicate your symptoms need further investigation. If you have one symptom such as mild pain for less than 24-hour and you went to the gym it is worth asking yourself is it a muscle strain? If you are able to be mindful of your symptoms and you notice there is more than one symptom of concern then seek medical advice. If you have all five symptoms of concern seek medical advice immediately especially if the symptom is alarming such as you are bleeding. Your doctor has probably given you a list of symptoms to be mindful of and watch out for in the future. If you don't have a list of things to be watching out for then ask, this will give you some idea of what you should and should not be concerned about. While no list of concerning symptoms can ever be exhaustive having some idea of what to look out for can possibly help you to feel more prepared.

3. **Impact on Well-Being:** The fear of cancer recurrence can have a profound impact on survivors' emotional, psychological, and social well-being. It may lead to heightened levels of anxiety, depression, hypervigilance regarding health, trouble concentrating or sleeping, avoidance of reminders of cancer, challenges with making future plans or commitments, and strained relationships with family and friends. If this is the case a number of your symptoms may be connected to trauma as a result of your diagnosis and treatment. If this is the case it may be that you need to get some further assistance to help you manage your symptoms. If you feel like your distress is impacting on your

relationships or you are not coping or you are struggling to get back into life you may be experiencing a trauma reaction.  We discussed the possibility of a trauma reaction at the beginning of the book but as I stated previously it may take some time for the distress to show up. While we often celebrate the end of treatment and everyone around us is also celebrating, the trauma associated with diagnosis and treatment is often underestimated. You may need to seek appropriate support to help you manage your symptoms you may also need mental health interventions to help get you back on track. This is why some people who have experienced cancer then suffer guilt because they don't feel "happy" once they have been given the all clear by their medical team. In fact people after treatment has finished may experience a decline in their mental health as they process all of the things that have just happened.

4. **Coping Strategies:** Coping with the fear of cancer recurrence involves developing strategies to manage anxiety and uncertainty while also living a fulfilling life. We have already talked a lot about coping skills and some of the strategies to help you manage are included in this book. Some other coping strategies include seeking support from healthcare providers, mental health professionals, and support groups for cancer survivors, practicing relaxation techniques such as deep breathing or mindfulness meditation, engaging in activities that promote self-care and well-being, maintaining a healthy lifestyle, regular exercise, balanced nutrition, and adequate sleep, and attending to what you can control rather than fixating on the possibility of recurrence.

5. **Helping others:** this is a personal choice and something that some people may feel uncomfortable about. However it can be of great value and great comfort to have someone who has been through treatment to connect with someone who is yet to start. It can be helpful to give some support to someone else who has recently been diagnosed and give them some strategies and some advice of what to expect particularly if there has been a similar diagnosis or treatment regime.   A similar experience can be very reassuring for someone especially if someone has found a way out the other side of cancer. Please be mindful that not everybody wants to connect with someone who has had cancer or even similar treatment but if the person is willing and seeks you out for advice this may be a positive experience for both you and for them. There is nothing more reassuring than meeting somebody who has gone into battle and won. It can also be helpful for people to hear that as you commence treatment there will be good days and bad days and also share in the funny experiences you may have engaged in along the way. It helps to demystify the treatment that is to come but also reassure the person that potentially with the right treatment and supports things can be okay.

By acknowledging and addressing the fear of cancer recurrence, survivors can take steps to manage their anxiety and live more fully in the present moment, while also remaining vigilant about their health and well-being.

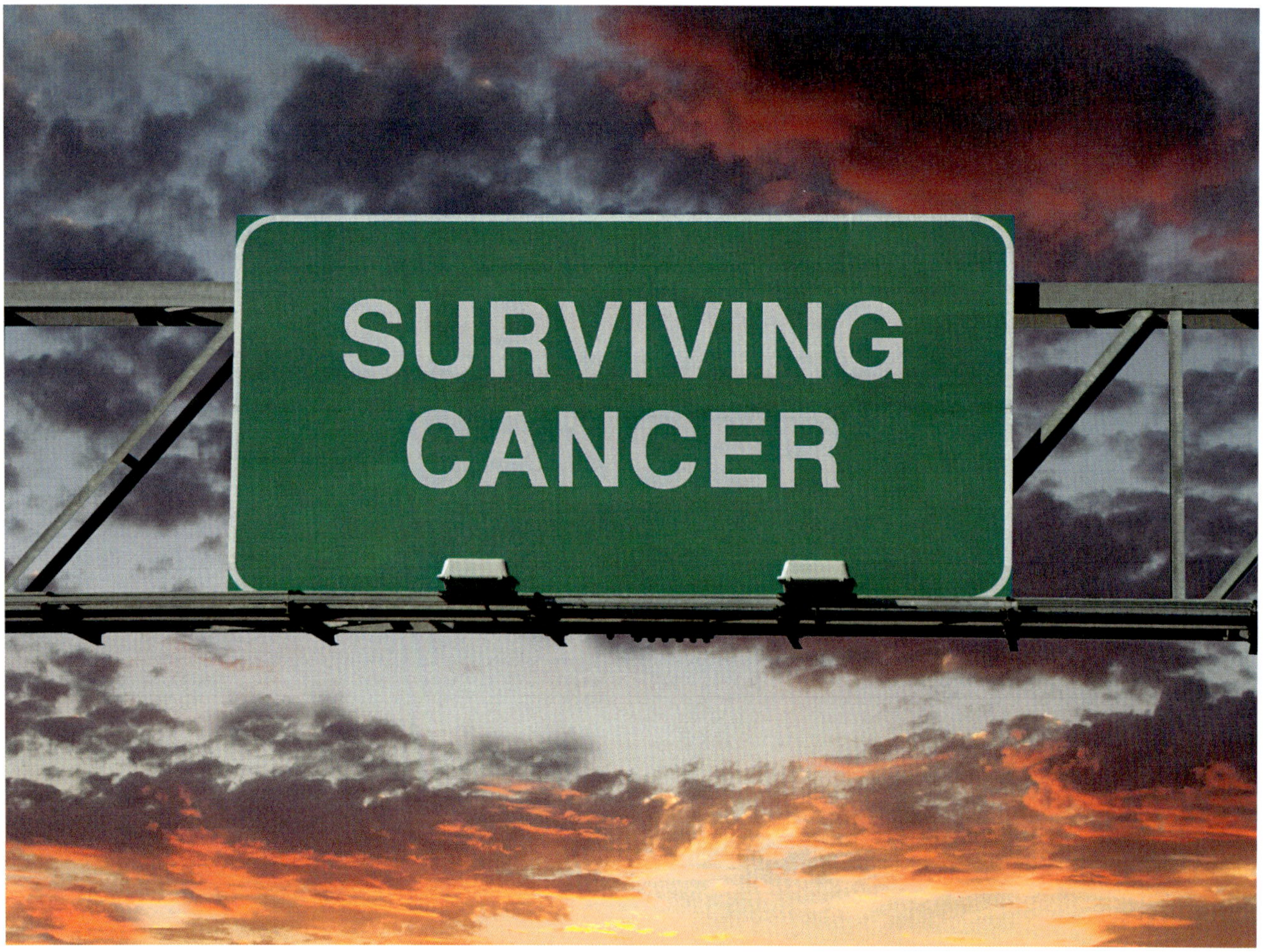

# LIVING WITH THE FEAR

Living with surviving a fatal illness presents unique challenges that require a blend of emotional, practical, social, spiritual, and cognitive strategies for acceptance and quality of life. While some of the strategies might seem repetitive the book is constructed to remind you of what to do and when. There will be different things that you need to consider at different stages of your journey. Here are some strategies that may help you to live with the fear:

**Emotional Strategies**

1. **Acknowledge Your Feelings:** Allow yourself to feel and express a wide range of emotions, such as anger, sadness, fear, and even joy. Keeping a journal or talking to a trusted friend or therapist can help process these emotions.
2. **Practice Self-Compassion:** Be kind to yourself and recognize that it's okay to have bad days. Treat yourself with the same compassion you would offer a loved one or friend in a similar situation.

**Practical Strategies**

1. **Educate Yourself:** Understanding your illness, treatment options, and prognosis can empower you to make informed decisions about your care.
2. **Advance Care Planning:** Make decisions about your future medical care, including advance directives, living wills, and designating a healthcare proxy.
3. **Manage Symptoms:** Work with your healthcare team to manage symptoms and improve your quality of life through medication, therapy, and lifestyle changes.

**Social Strategies**

1. **Build a Support Network:** Surround yourself with supportive family, friends, and healthcare providers who can offer emotional and practical help. Seek out others who can be constructive rather than focus on the negatives.
2. **Communicate Openly:** Keep open lines of communication with your loved ones about your needs, feelings, and wishes. Honest conversations can strengthen relationships and provide mutual support.
3. **Join Support Groups or find others who share your experience:** Connecting with other people who are facing similar challenges can provide a sense of community, understanding, and shared experiences. Make sure these are people who are in a good place and you are not opening yourself up to be a support for someone who is a bit emotionally fragile and who will only make things worse. You don't want to end up supporting someone else which might make you very vulnerable.

**Spiritual Strategies**

1. **Explore Spiritual Practices:** Engage in spiritual or religious practices that bring

you comfort, such as prayer, meditation, or attending religious services. This is not for everyone but you might find it is very helpful and connects you to a whole new group of people.

2. **Seek Meaning:** Reflect on your beliefs, values, and the meaning of life. Finding purpose in daily activities, relationships, and personal growth can provide solace. This happens a lot! People can really re-evaluate their lives after going through something difficult and it can make them re-focus on what is important. People have been known to change jobs, careers, re-evaluate relationships and also what brings them joy and leave things that make them unhappy. You won't be the first or last person to make major life changes after surviving cancer.

### Cognitive Strategies

1. **Focus on the Present:** Practice mindfulness and stay present in the moment. Techniques such as deep breathing, meditation, and mindful activities can help reduce anxiety about the future.
2. **Radical Acceptance:** This is when we accept the situation (and no we don't have to like it) but then we can find solutions. If we are fighting something we are resisting and unlikely to be able to not only not process emotions but we are fighting the reality. Unfortunately it is what it is.
3. **Set Realistic Goals:** Establish achievable goals that bring you joy and a sense of accomplishment, whether they are daily tasks or long-term aspirations. you might take up some other hobbies as a result or decide to learn to play the instrument that you have always put off until now. Alternatively you may also decide to set goals around fitness and health building up slowly. You are unlikely to be able to jump straight back into life as it was before but setting goals and then achieving them can help build confidence.
4. **Reframe Your Thoughts:** Challenge negative thoughts and try to reframe them in a more positive or realistic light. Cognitive-behavioural therapy (CBT) techniques can be particularly helpful. We have discussed these earlier in the book. Refer back to these strategies and put them into practice as you are learning to live with the fear of recurrence.

### Quality of Life Strategies

1. **Engage in Enjoyable Activities:** Continue to pursue hobbies and activities that bring you pleasure and a sense of normalcy. Go enjoy life, spend time with family, friends, your dog! Go do things that make you happy and take pleasure in the small things that a few months ago may have seemed very out of reach.
2. **Maintain Routine:** Keeping a regular routine can provide structure and a sense of control in your daily life. Start off small maybe begin with the basics such as doing the washing, then build up to more ambitious things such as cleaning

the house or building up your exercise from 10 mins to 30 mins at the same time every day.

3. **Focus on Self-Care:** Prioritize activities that promote your physical, emotional, and mental well-being, such as exercise, healthy eating, and relaxation techniques. You can now focus on helping your body recover and doing everything that you can to stay well.

Acceptance and adaptation are ongoing processes. It's essential to find what works best for you and to seek support when needed.

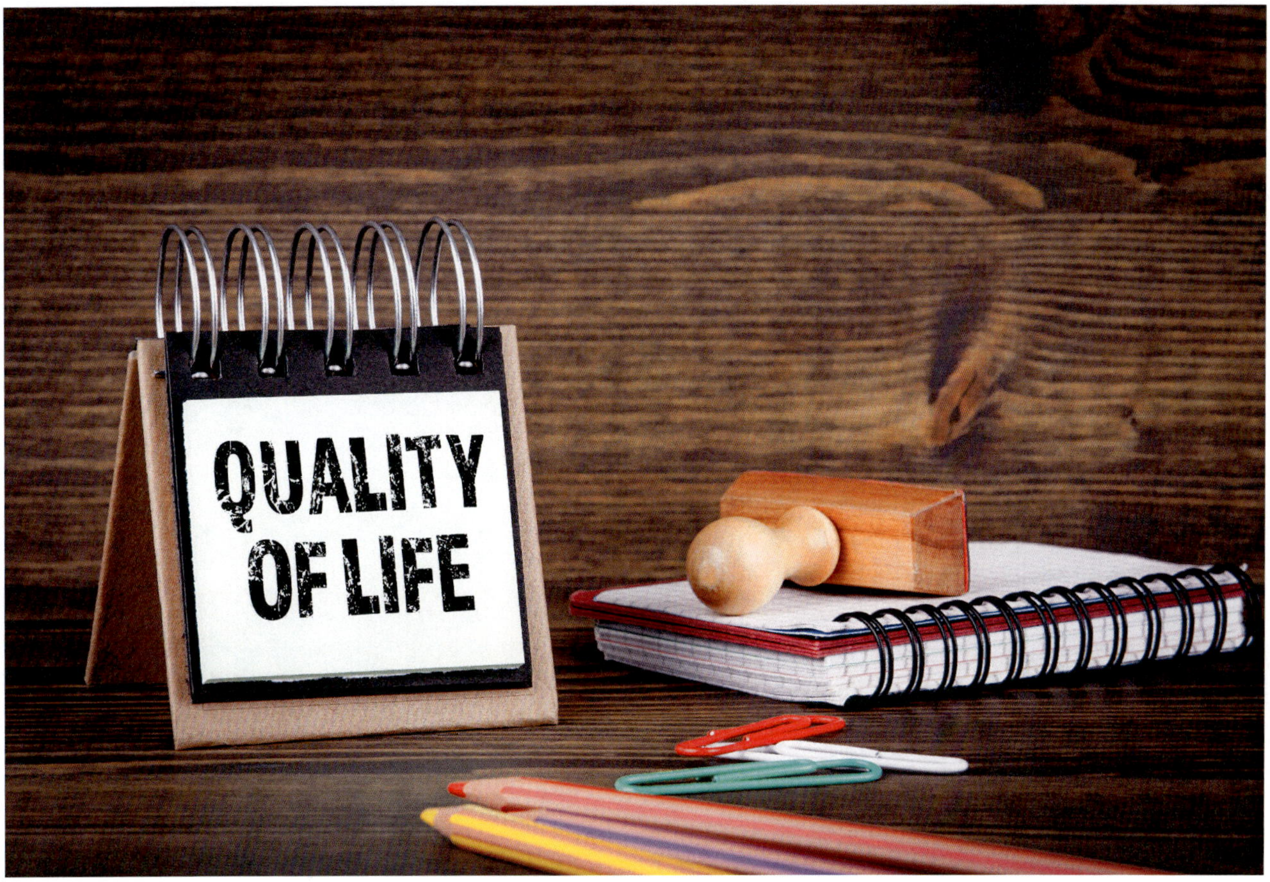

# ONLY OPEN AND WORK ON THIS SECTION WHEN YOU NEED TOO.

# SEALED SECTION

This is the section you read and work on when you are ready or if you have to. There are no "should" to be followed. I debated about this section and including it as the last thing I want to think about for anyone suffering is that there is not a good outcome. When discussing this book with others and what should be included I was surprised how many people said that it was important as a section as it "helped" them have a sense of control over the choices they might need to make. Only look at this bit if you need or want to and everyone is different. This is the section that you read when you have a cup of tea in your hand and it is time to plan. You will know in yourself if the things in this section will be applicable to you. This is not an exhaustive list of things that you might need to consider but, like the rest of the book each section is a series of things that you might want to consider. Be gentle with yourself and maybe do this bit over a few days if you feel like it is a bit confronting.

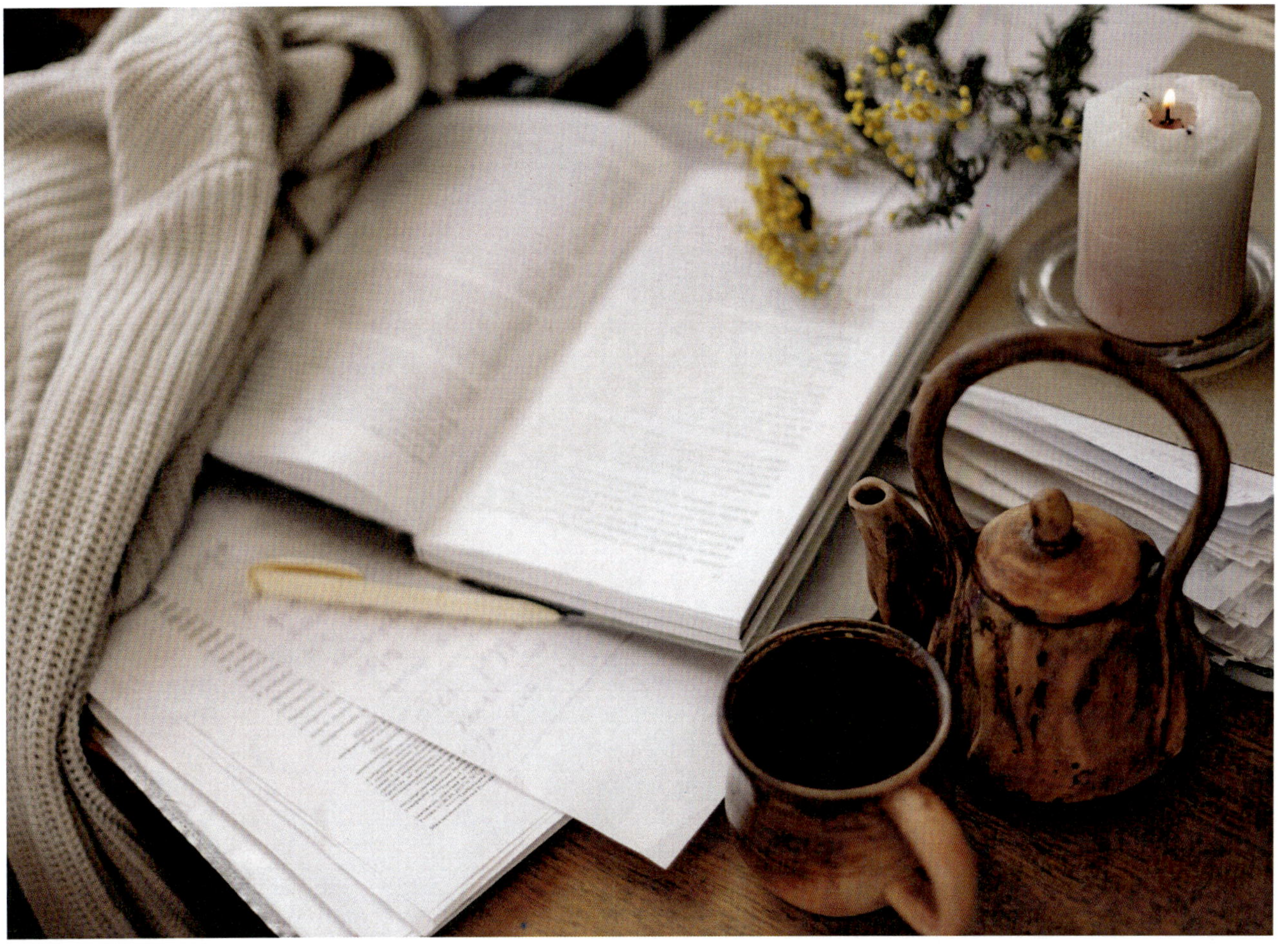

# PLANNING

Ok so now you have been given the news from your medical team that things may result in a different outcome. Treatment has either become palliative or you want to be prepared. I am sorry and I wish it could be different. If you are looking at this section you have taken the time to sit with your thoughts, you are ready to plan for either your passing or you want to be prepared in case you are unable to put things in place because you are too unwell. Organising the end of a life is actually very time consuming and if you are reading this you are wanting to think about the things you might need to be aware of. Further, you may also want to consider how you can organise things to help your family who will be grieving if you have passed on. You may also want to have some control over the way you are remembered by those who knew you or cared for you. This section will be difficult but take the time and if you need to take it to your therapist or advisors to discuss important key points. There are sections to write notes if you want to, or you can come back and fill in these sections as you need to. Alternatively, you may just want to have some ideas in the back of your head in case things need to be considered.

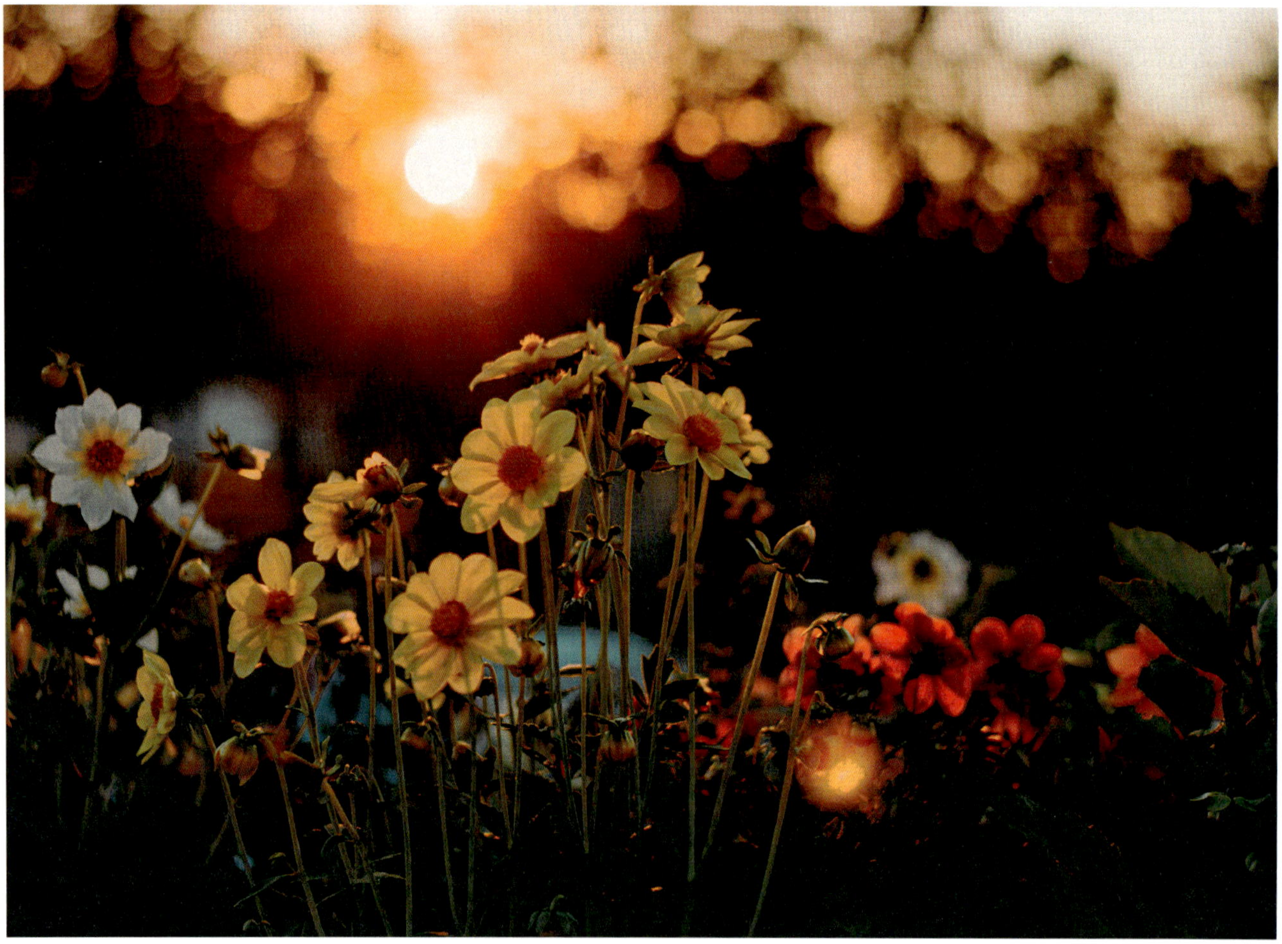

# END OF LIFE CHOICES

If you are preparing for the end of your life when you have cancer then this is a deeply personal time that involves emotional, practical, personal and medical considerations. This section is to help you continue to have some choices over what happens to you and to help you put in place things that are going to make you feel like you have some control over this stage of your life. Here are some things that it is important for you to consider:

**Emotional and Psychological Preparation:**

1. **Open Communication:**
   - Talk openly with your family and friends about your feelings, fears, and wishes. Honest conversations can help everyone involved to prepare. Yes everyone is going to be upset and there are going to be lots of emotions. You can also ask for what you want from others such as "just be normal with me" or "make me laugh", "treat me as normal". This is the time to ask and be a bit selfish after all it is about you. Not everyone wants to see people grieving them before they are actually gone but be realistic while some are able to hold it together for a period of time they might also "lose it" on occasions. If you find this hard ask them to perhaps leave the room or stay away for a few days if you find it too difficult. You get to ask for what you need right now is about you!
   - Consider discussing your wishes for your final days, such as where you want to be (at home, in a hospice, etc.) and who you want to be with you. This might be hard for children or close family who will want to be there for you. They might find it very difficult and for children hospitals can be very confronting places. Seek out your special humans and talk about what you want. You may also only want a few people to come and visit you in your final stages, not a cast of thousands. Maybe have a check list of who is allowed and who might be a definite "NO". You may also want to consider your pets or animals (of the fur variety) and how you are going to manage this towards the end. Do you want them to visit or do you want them close (on the bed). They are possibly grieving you too and being close can be a comfort.

2. **Counselling and Support Groups:**
   - Find a good therapist if you haven't found one already. A therapist may help you to think about what you want. Also sometimes it is difficult to be honest with your partner or close friends it can be easier to speak to someone who is a professional and then you can "leave it in the therapy room" and go as best as you can about your day. One of the hardest things is to say out loud the difficult things and then to face your loved one who is also facing their own fears around your health. If you get a therapist then ensure they are right one for you if not, don't be afraid to find another. This happens all the time and as a therapist let me reassure you if we are not a good fit then I won't take it personally if you find someone else. A lot of therapy practices have more than one therapist attached to them and you have to find someone you can relate to

to discuss these important matters.

Working with people who are facing death is a very profound experience and I can honestly say that I have valued every one of those experiences. I have also as a therapist had to put aside what I thought "end of life" therapy would look like and "go with the flow". I think the hardest part is watching someone reconcile leaving loved ones behind and fearing they will be forgotten or they won't be missed which is simply never the case. You will be missed, never doubt that!

It is also hard to let someone work through issues and still find humour in the darkest moments. One lovely man I worked with years ago brought his wife to one of his final sessions and solemnly explained to her that he wanted her to re-partner after he died. Although they had been married for three decades he told her that she was "free to re-partner" with either a man or woman! He thought his comments were hilarious and he promptly burst into laughter....she did not find his comments funny and told him "once was enough". The look she gave him could have frozen Vodka! He died a couple of weeks later and to the best of my knowledge his wife has not re-partnered but he felt that he had given his wife permission to get on with her life, which he thought was important and gave him peace.

3. **Spiritual Care:**
   - If you have religious or spiritual beliefs, connect with a chaplain, clergy member, or spiritual advisor for support and guidance. Not everyone has a faith but as you might be approaching the end of your life it might be something you feel you have a need to do. That's ok. Find someone who you think will be supportive and consider why you have chosen to reach out. Is it to ask questions about the afterlife or is it for another reason?
   - Engage in spiritual practices that bring you peace, such as prayer, meditation, or reading spiritual texts. You might also find comfort in other things such as books about a spiritual subject. Either way do what works for you.
   - You may also have other ways to achieve these things such as through journaling or Art or even just being in a special place. There is no one way to find spiritual care or engage in the practice.

## To do list

# LEGAL/FINANCIAL CHOICES

I am not a lawyer but here are some things that you might want to consider. These are ideas and suggestions but if you are in doubt reach out to a lawyer who specialises in estates. As a therapist I have witnessed over the years so much distress over an estate as a legal will was not left for family to abide by. This situation causes so much unnecessary heartbreak and distress for those who loved you and might be grieving.

**Practical and Legal Preparation:**

1. **Advance Directives:**
   - Create an advance directive, which includes a living will and a durable power of attorney for healthcare. This document outlines your wishes for medical treatment and appoints someone to make decisions on your behalf if you are unable to do so.
   - Clearly state your preferences regarding life-sustaining treatments, pain management, and other medical interventions.

2. **Last Will and Testament:**
   - Ensure you have a valid will that outlines how you want your assets and possessions to be distributed after your passing. Make sure it is with a lawyer and also make sure your family know it exists. Far too many times a Will is found in a drawer or the family are totally unaware of its existence. Let someone know where your will is and how to find it, or the legal firm it is with. Save everyone the headache of playing the guessing game of "where is the will"? Trust me it is not a fun game!
   - Be mindful of changing your will multiple times.....it is your will but if you feel pressured to make changes as you near the end then this can cause havoc after you have passed. No one has the right to pressure you into making changes when you are at the end stage of your life. Also changing your will in the last few days of you life will only cause distress in the family. Be mindful of this.
   - Consider including any personal messages or letters to loved ones.
   - If you are also leaving behind younger children you may want to leave messages for them as they age or video messages about the things you would like to say as they get older. These might include messages for their wedding day or the day they have their first child. You may also want to leave some gifts for special days.
   - Find a good lawyer who can help you with this who is experienced in this area. Once your will is done you don't need to worry and you can focus on spending time on what is important to you in your time left.
   - Not all families are nice and some of you will have tricky family situations. Take the time to sit down and carefully plan out how you want your assets to be distributed and to whom. Further, also be aware that extended family comes out of the woodwork at a time like this so be careful about changing your will at the last minute and creating confusion. If you choose to change things then that is fine and your choice...Just be mindful that sometimes people do not always have your best interests at heart.

3. **Financial and Legal Affairs:**
   - Organize important documents, such as insurance policies, bank statements, and property deeds. Make sure your designated executor or power of attorney has access to these documents. Ensure that these are all in one place and can be easily found. Your grieving family are not going to have the emotional strength to track down all the bits of paper and it is going to be their job to close accounts, and sell assets if needed. Therefore, it might be a good idea to put all of your important documents in a folder probably labelled "Important Documents". Yes it is obvious but I bet people still ask where the key bits of info are!

4. **Funeral and Memorial Planning:**
   - Plan your funeral or memorial service according to your wishes. Decide on details such as the type of service, location, music, readings, and any special requests. What the flowers might be? The photos you want as part of your tribute. You might also want to consider how you want to be dressed? Other things you might want to consider are an open or closed casket? Cremation? Burial? Do you want to be composted...apparently that it is thing now.....or do you want to become a gem stone? Or go into the sky as a firework? Think about what you might like and then find out what is possible. You may meet some resistance especially for the more unusual suggestions or ideas you might have, but this is your moment.
   - Also consider if you would like a wake and where you would like that to be. Do you want it catered? This can be very important to some people to have a chance to de-brief after the funeral service and share stories about you. Sometimes funeral houses have a function centre connected to the funeral home and they can organise catering. If not consider who would have the capacity to organise a wake and if others contribute food or if it is not catered for.
   - Also consider the size of your funeral do you want it to be a small affair or allow anyone to attend. This will also impact on catering and the venue.
   - Also consider if there are people who you do not want to attend your funeral. This is your moment and you get to choose.
   - It might be important to find a funeral house and start discussing what your end of life experience might be. Perhaps make an appointment and take a support person with you to help you make these decisions. Making these decisions after you are gone is difficult for your family or loved ones and they may be very overwhelmed to try and think about what you might like or how you would like to be remembered. When my grandmother died at the ripe old age of 99....of old age...we had no idea what she wanted for her funeral. I happened to be looking through her old Bible and found some ideas and also found out that her name wasn't even the one she was born with...she just decided she hated her name and gave herself a new one! These are the sorts of things that family has to deal with after your passing. Try to not make the process harder than it needs to be.
   - Write down your requests so that your family or loved ones are able to easily

carry out and respect your wishes rather than be confused or do what they think is best. Remember they are not always going to be thinking clearly at this time.

- Communicate your preferences to your family or designated representative.

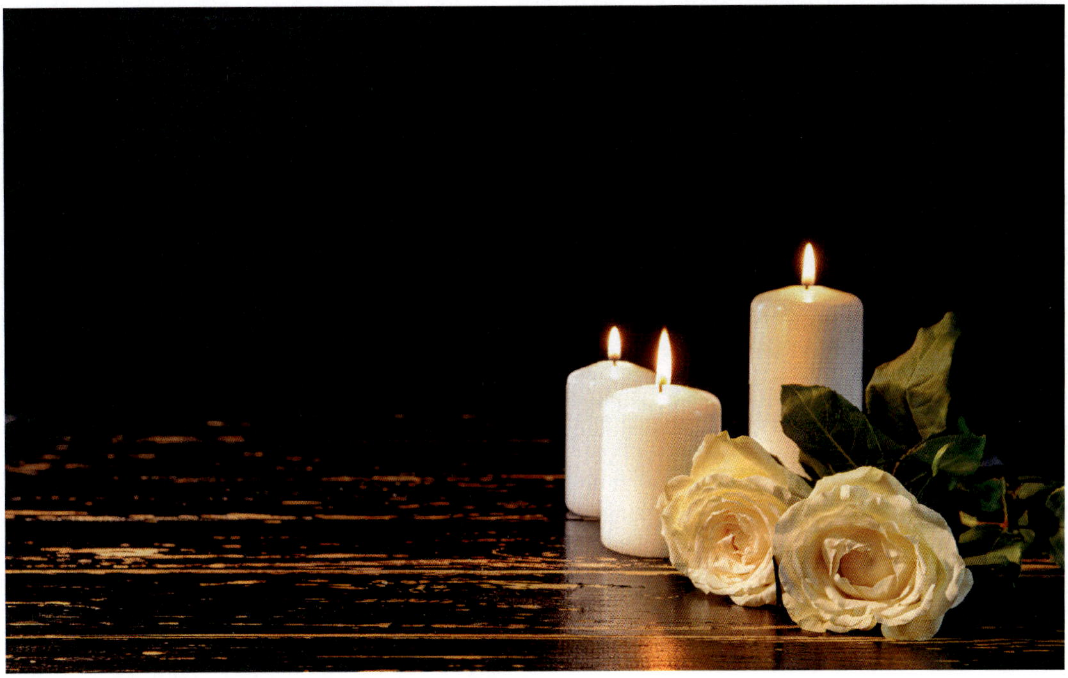

## To do list

# MEDICAL CHOICES

You have some things to consider here and take time to think about what you might want:

**Medical and Physical Preparation:**

1. **Palliative Care:**
    - Engage with a Palliative care team (there will be one in your local area) to manage symptoms and improve your quality of life. Palliative care focuses on relief from pain and other distressing symptoms and to help you feel more physically comfortable as you near the end of your life. At the Palliative stage it is mostly about pain management.
    - Make the time to discuss how palliative care can be organised and how this can help you.
    - Will you be able to stay at home or will you need to go to hospital? This might depend on your medical condition and who might be able to look after you.
    - How long will you be able to receive care at home?
    - What will that look like? Will you be eligible for nursing care?
    - Discuss your goals of care with your healthcare team, including your preferences for comfort measures and any specific treatments you want or do not want.

1. **Hospice Care:**
    - Consider enrolling in hospice care if your prognosis indicates that you are nearing the end of life. Hospice care provides comprehensive support for you and your family, focusing on comfort and quality of life rather than curative treatments.
    - Hospice services can be provided at home, in a hospice facility, or in a hospital. Find out from your medical team what might be available and how this can be accessed.

## To do list

# FAMILY AND LOVED ONES

This is a tough section and one that is going to be hard for you and those who love you.

**Family and Loved Ones:**

1. **Communication and Support:**
    - Keep your family and loved ones informed about your condition and your wishes. Encourage them to ask questions and express their feelings.
    - Consider involving them in caregiving tasks if they are willing and able, but also be mindful of their limits and encourage them to seek support.
    - Also as I have already spoken about consider how you would like friends and family to treat you towards the end. Do you want them to try and carry on as normal and just talk about rubbish with you? Both of you know that things are difficult but are you the sort of person who wants to focus on the negatives or positives? Is it important to you to laugh and make memories and will talking about it only make you more scared or worried? Everyone is different but having a think might help you to be prepared. Also you have every right to change your mind!

2. **Legacy and Remembrance:**
    - Create opportunities to share memories, stories, and experiences with your loved ones. Consider writing letters, making recordings, or creating memory books. One great idea I heard about was a book of recipes of favourite foods that a mother organised for each of her children. This was clearly meaningful and had such a lot of love behind it. Other things to consider is if you want to leave certain things to certain people such as gifts to friends that might have special meaning for you both. Maybe ask as there is no point leaving someone a BBQ when they have one and yours is falling apart. A photo of the two of you might have more meaning.
    - Discuss ways you would like to be remembered and any specific legacies you want to leave behind.

3. **Conflict:**
    - Be careful about people close to you suddenly making it difficult for your family to see you, isolating you and it is very destructive. Take control of who you want to see and be mindful of those who speak negatively about your children or family.
    - If there is family conflict, this is a time when you would hope everyone pulls together but not necessarily so. If there are issues within the family then it might be a good idea to sit everyone down and explain what you want. Your children are your children and your partner is your partner.

- Try to keep it simple and for goodness sake don't let people keep people away from you at this time, unless there is a **VERY** good reason. Personally I can't think of a good enough reason to be prevented from seeing someone you love when you are dying. This behaviour should give off **VERY LARGE ALARM BELLS!**
- If someone who claims to care about you is doing this sort of behaviour they perhaps have an agenda and this is never good.
- Also it is important to remember that there are all sorts of families out there. Marriages end, people re-partner, people also have a second family or more children. Consider that when you re-partner do not just "wipe" people from your lives such as children from your first marriage because your new "wife" who you met recently on a Cruise Ship thinks this is a great idea! Yes it happens.....Just because she is telling you she/he/they will look after you and they are 15 years younger is not a reason to suddenly change your Will excluding those who love you and have put up with you for a lot longer than your new partner! While this sounds like a good idea in theory it is not respectful to your children or grandchildren and is very, very hurtful to those who love you. Also making the statement to yourself "well I can do what I want and I won't need to worry I will be dead!" is just not going to cut it. That is very much a "cop out". You are going to really hurt a lot of people who love you with that attitude. Be fair to your new partner but also be fair to your children and loved ones.
- Carefully consider your actions as I promise you this is the stuff of challenging Wills and families going to court and the only people who win are the lawyers as they get paid a fortune once people start arguing!
- If you have a complex family situation then sit down with key people and explain your Will prior to your death. This will alleviate (hopefully) any reasons for tension after you are gone. In my experience people don't go to court to fight over something stupid after someone has passed on, they challenge a Will because they are hurt and you have possibly disrespected them in your final moments. You may have made decisions when you are not thinking clearly and you are scared and vulnerable. People end up challenging a Will due to money/assets being left to a new partner which then is left to their family, (not return to your family or children) if they should pass on. Do you really want your hard earned money to go to some "weird cousin" of your new partner? Further, if this cousin or relative lives off the grid they can then give your hard earned money to the cat home as opposed to your grandchildren who actually knew you?
- As a "biological relative" your children can challenge your Will if you do not carefully consider the possible outcomes and plan for the unexpected.
- Be smart if there are complex family dynamics and consider getting some very good advice regarding your Will and how it can be set up and consider all the options. Most people go into this area blind to what the outcomes can be. This is where we really see the good the bad and the **REALLY** ugly!

# SELF CARE

**Look After you......**

**Self-Care and Comfort:**

1. **Pain and Symptom Management:**
   - Work closely with your healthcare team to manage pain and other symptoms effectively. Do not hesitate to communicate any changes or concerns about your comfort.
   - Use medications, therapies, and complementary approaches (such as massage, acupuncture, or aromatherapy) as recommended.

2. **Personal Comfort:**
   - Surround yourself with items and activities that bring you comfort and joy, such as favourite music, books, or hobbies.
   - Create a peaceful and comfortable environment in your home or care setting.
   - Do what you enjoy, which might be walking or sitting in your garden every day in the sun.
   - Look at photos or watch shows that you enjoy.
   - Make a commitment to yourself to ensure quality of life and this means only doing what you enjoy. I used to have a lovely elderly man in my neighbourhood who walked every day with his daughter. I started to wonder why at about the same time every day my big shaggy Golden Retriever Gracie would be waiting patiently at the front fence. I eventually caught him giving Gracie a biscuit. He told me "I know I'm not supposed to feed your dog but I have cancer and so you have to let me". I agreed and told him that it sounded reasonable to me and that who was I to deny him...or the dog. Gracie waited every day for her "friend" to come past the gate with her head hanging out of the fence looking in the direction he would walk up the street for her biscuit and pat . This gentleman did this ritual daily until eventually he passed away a few months later. Gracie waited for her friend at the fence for months at the same time every day even after he had passed on. His daughter later told me it was always the highlight of her father's walk and it made him very happy.

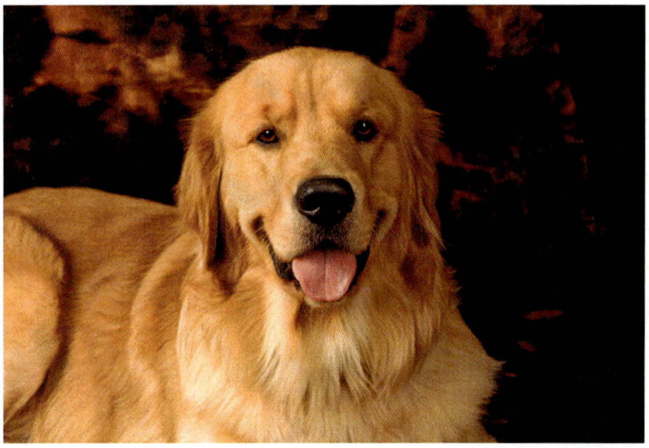

# A FINAL WORD

Preparing for the end of life when you have cancer involves addressing emotional, practical, and medical needs. Open communication, careful planning, and seeking appropriate support can help you and your loved ones navigate this difficult time with dignity and peace. By taking these steps, you can ensure that your wishes are respected, your affairs are in order, and your remaining time is spent in the most meaningful and comfortable way possible rather than leaving behind a big fat mess for others to clean up. Your family want to remember you with fond memories not anger and frustration and more hurt than is necessary. This is not a time in your life to play games or use this as an opportunity to seek revenge on others. This won't bring you peace and it certainly won't help your family.
Thank you for reading this book and I hope it has helped you in some small way. The book was created to help people like you find a way through what ever the outcome. This book is not intended to be an authority on the subject of Cancer but rather some ideas and suggestions to help you make the next stages of coping with your diagnosis and treatment more bearable.

I have made the decision to donate to Cancer research a portion of the proceeds of each of the guidebooks sold. So you are not only helping yourself by working through this book but you are also helping others.

I wish you all the best and genuinely hope you find a way out to the other side. Take care of yourself and those around you.

Oh and good luck!

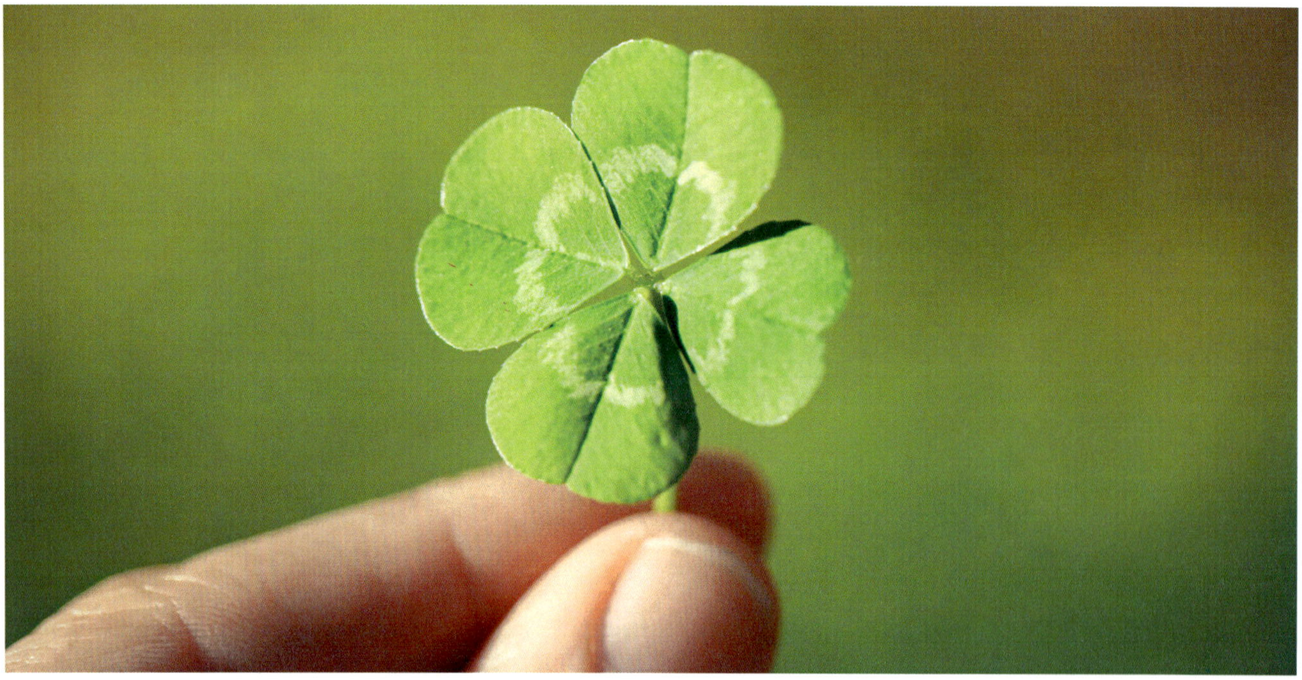

*YOUR GO TO*

# RESOURCE LIST

SUPPORT GORUPS

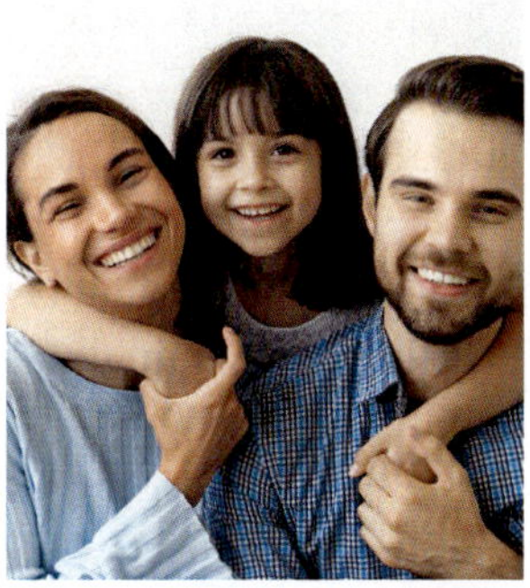

FACEBOOK GROUPS

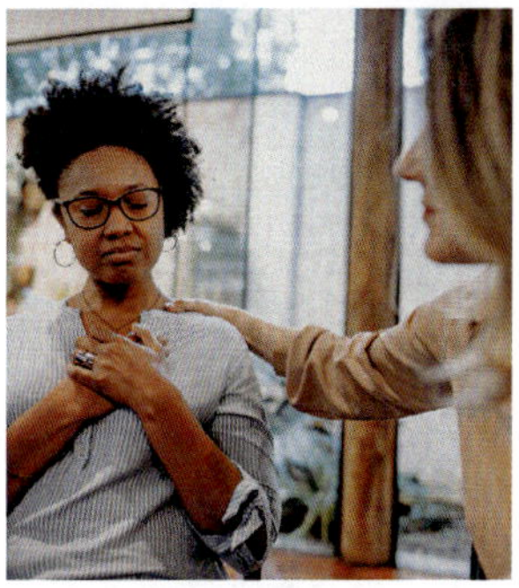

OTHER

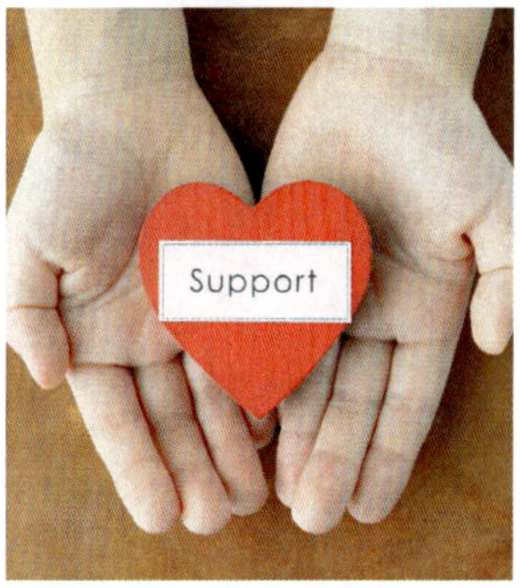


OTHER

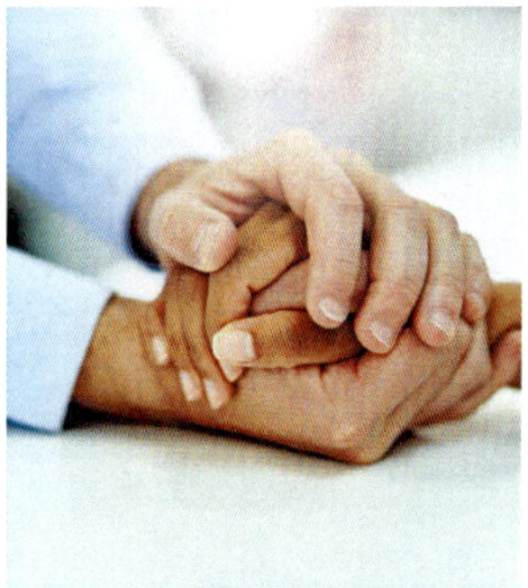

The future is unwritten..........

You can survive and thrive......

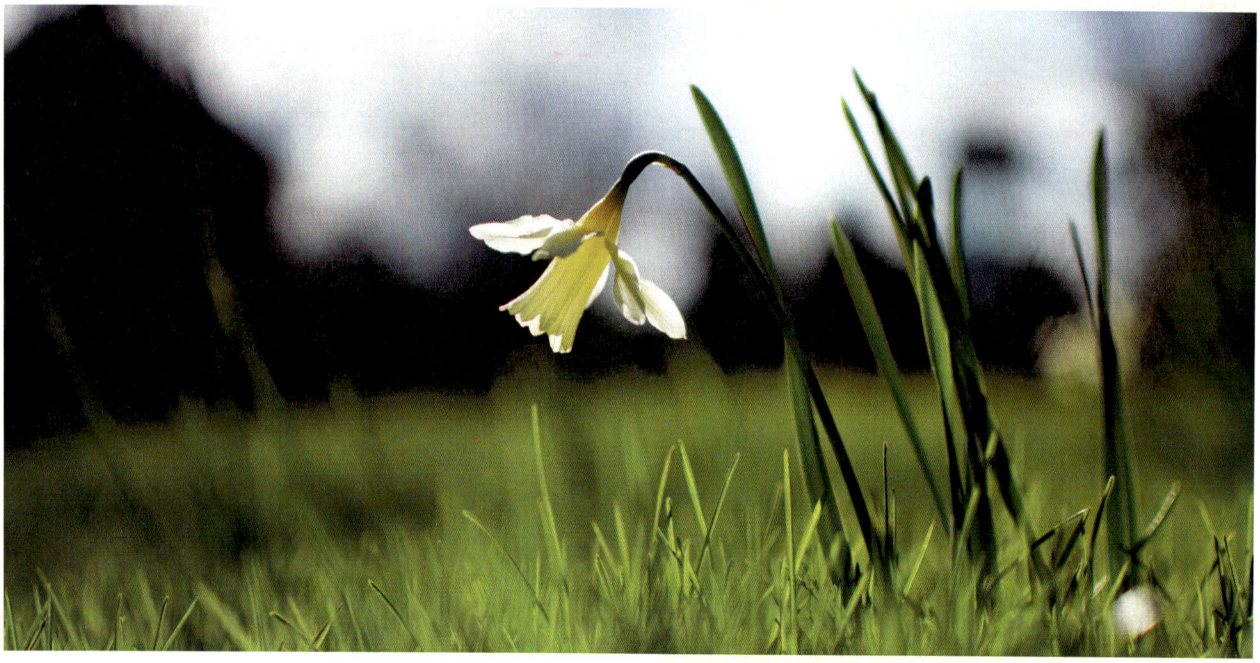

## References

Beck, A. T. (1963). Thinking and depression: I. Idiosyncratic content and cognitive distortions. Archives of General Psychiatry, 9, 324-333. DOI: 10.1001/archpsyc.1963.01720160014002.

Beck, J. S. (2011). Cognitive behaviour therapy: Basics and beyond (2nd ed.). Guilford Press.

Bowlby, J. (1969). Attachment. New York: Basic Books.

Cancer Council Australia

Crufad.org (2010) Posttraumatic Stress Disorder, Patient treatment Manual. St Vincent's Hospital Sydney.

Knauss, C., & Schofield, M.J. (2009). A resource for counsellors and psychotherapists working with clients suffering from posttraumatic stress disorder. Melbourne: PACFA.

Linehan, M., M., (2014). DBT Training Manual. New York, NY: The Guilford Press.

G Taylor EMDR Therapist Training Manual Schema Therapy Training online

C. Van Woudenberg, E. M. Voorendonk, H. Bongaerts, H. A. Zoet, M. Verhagen, C. W. Lee, A. van Minnen & A. De Jongh (2018) Effectiveness of an intensive treatment programme combining prolonged exposure and eye movement desensitization and reprocessing for severe post-traumatic stress disorder, European Journal of Psychotraumatology, 9:1, DOI: 10.1080/20008198.2018.1487225

https://www.cancer.org/cancer/end-of-life-care/nearing-the-end-of-life/planning.html

Understanding PTSD and PTSD treatment
https://www.ptsd.va.gov/understand/what/index.asp

Vora, E., & Stevens, E. (2022). The anatomy of anxiety: understanding and overcoming the body's fear response. Unabridged. [United States], Harper Collins Publishers.

# WORKSHEETS

# TO DO LIST

*Make a list of things you need to consider:*

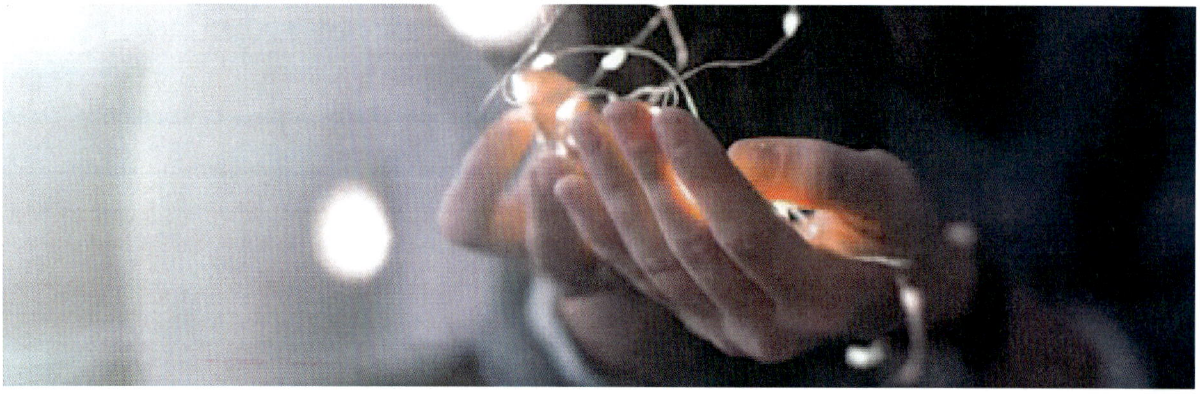

# WRITE YOURSELF A LETTER

Dear ______________________

I wanted to take a moment to thank you for our wonderful life together. Looking back, I'm glad we got it done.

We did the best thing we've ever done.

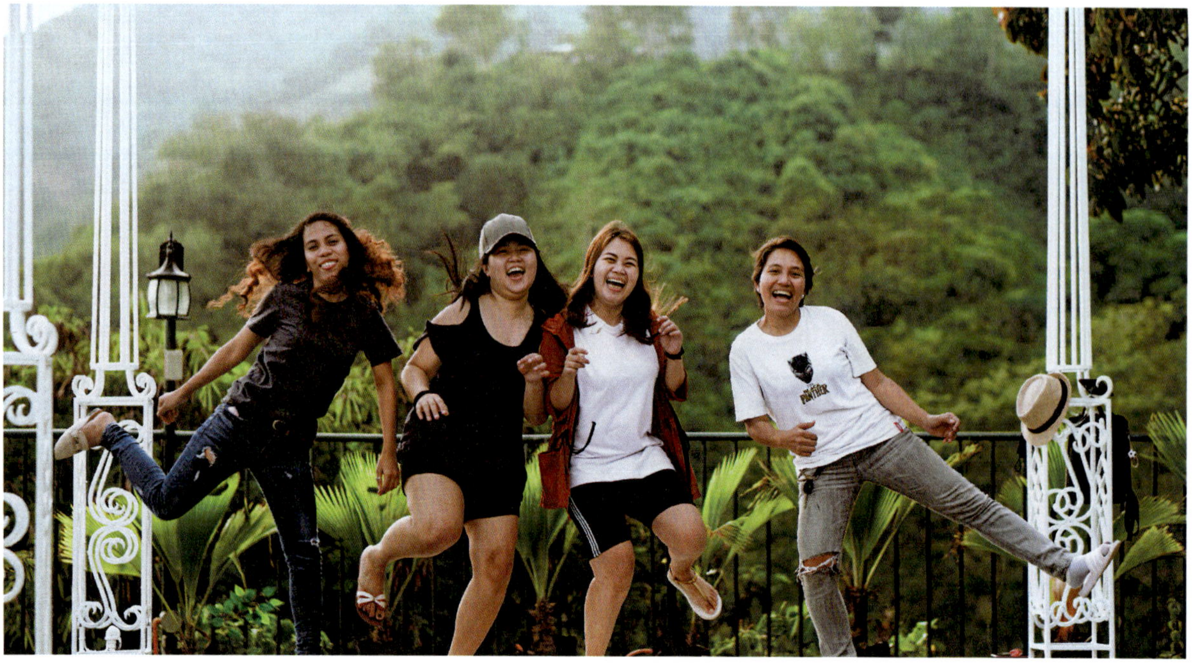

# LAUGHTER IS THE MOST EFFECTIVE MEDICINE

When was the last time you had a good laugh?

What caused you to laugh?

What TV show makes you laugh the most?

Who in your family or circle of friends makes you laugh?

You'll feel silly, but fake a laugh for effect.

*In 30 seconds your seritonin levels will rise...*

What is important to you...

What do you value? Someone once said we value what we would rescue in a fire.

# WHAT MAKES YOU FEEL STRONG?

# WHAT GIVES YOU A SENSE OF CONTROL?

# TAKE A LOOK OUT YOUR WINDOW...

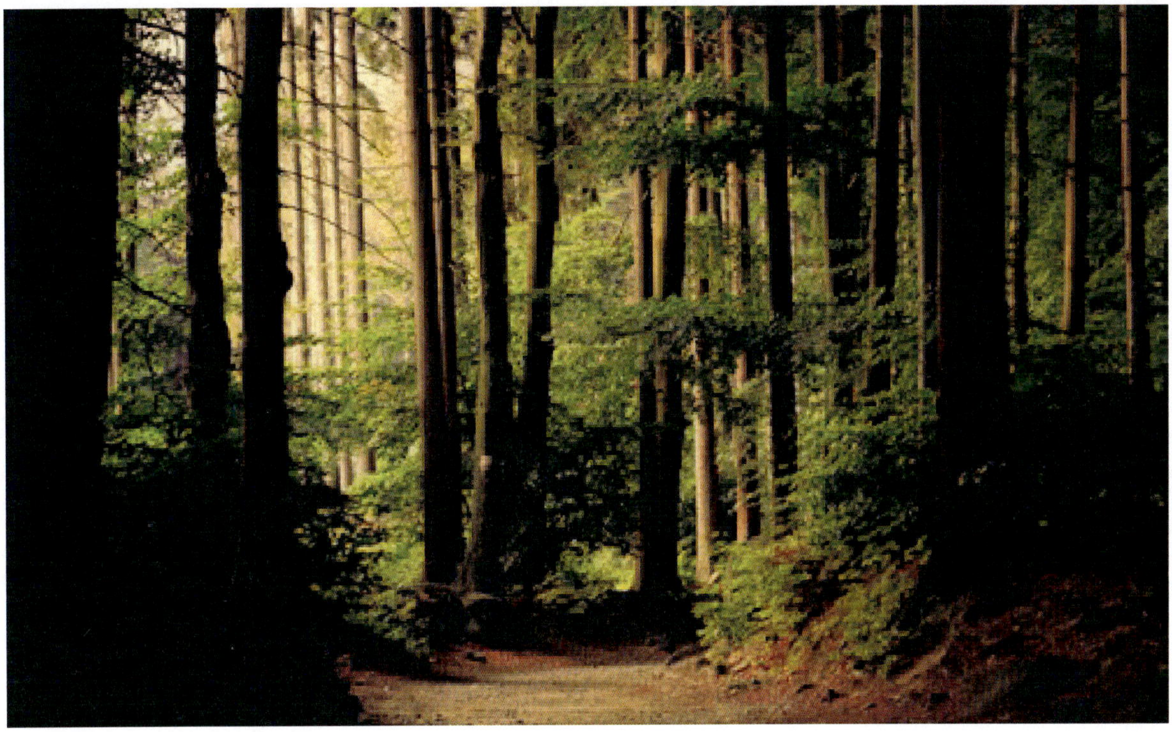

*What do you notice?*
***LIST EVERY DETAIL!*** *This is good brain exercise!*

# THINGS THAT ARE DISTRACTING FROM BAD THOUGHTS

1.

2.

3.

4.

5.

6.

7.

8.

9.

10.

11.

12.

# TIPS

## WHAT'S THE BEST PIECE OF ADVICE YOU'VE EVER RECEIVED?

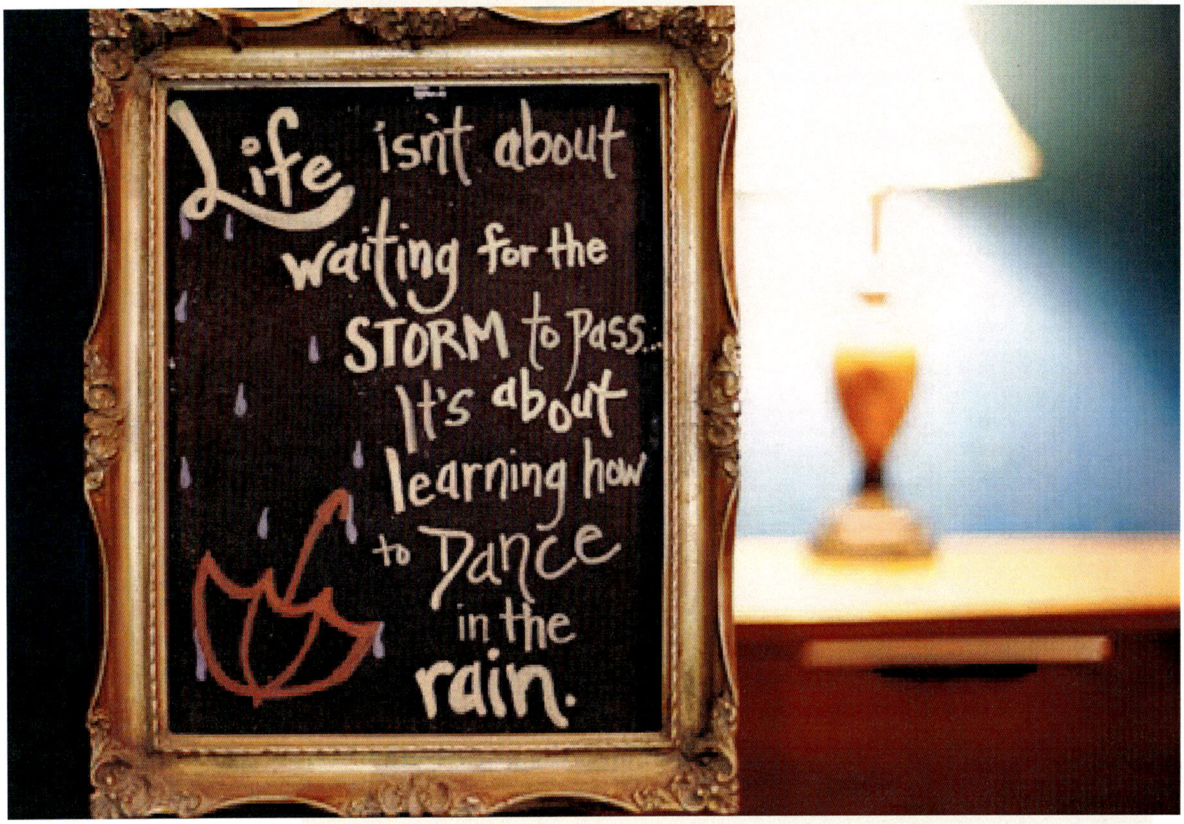

# NOTES SPACE

# NOTES SPACE

# NOTES SPACE

# NOTES SPACE

# NOTES SPACE

# NOTES SPACE

# NOTES SPACE

# NOTES SPACE

# NOTES SPACE

# NOTES SPACE

# NOTES SPACE

# NOTES SPACE

# NOTES SPACE

# NOTES SPACE

# NOTES SPACE

# NOTES SPACE

# NOTES SPACE

# NOTES SPACE

# NOTES SPACE

# NOTES SPACE

# NOTES SPACE

# NOTES SPACE